Making Sense of Death, Dying and Bereavement

Making Sense of Death, Dying and Bereavement: An Anthology

This Anthology, along with the companion volume *Death and Dying: A Reader* edited by Sarah Earle, Carol Komaromy and Caroline Bartholomew, form part of the Open University course Death and Dying (K260), a 30 point second level undergraduate course. The course forms part of the BA/BSc (Hons) in Health Studies, the BA/BSc (Hons) in Health and Social Care and the BA/BSc (Hons) in Social Work.

Details of this and other Open University courses can be obtained from the Student Registration and Enquiry Service, The Open University, PO Box 197, Milton Keynes MK7 6BJ, United Kingdom, tel. +44 (0)845 300 6090, e-mail general-enquiries@open.ac.uk

Alternatively, you may visit the Open University website at http://www.open.ac.uk where you can learn more about the wide range of courses and packs offered at all levels by The Open University.

Making Sense of Death, Dying and Bereavement

An Anthology

Edited by
Sarah Earle, Caroline Bartholomew and Carol Komaromy

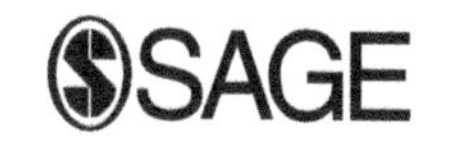

Los Angeles | London | New Delhi
Singapore | Washington DC

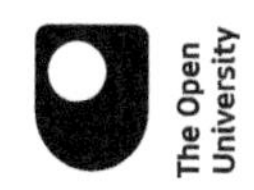

First published 2009

SAGE Publications Ltd
1 Oliver's Yard
55 City Road
London EC1Y 1SP

SAGE Publications Inc.
2455 Teller Road
Thousand Oaks, California 91320

SAGE Publications India Pvt Ltd
B 1/I 1 Mohan Cooperative Industrial Area
Mathura Road
New Delhi 110 044

SAGE Publications Asia-Pacific Pte Ltd
3 Church Street
#10-04 Samsung Hub
Singapore 049483

Library of Congress Control Number: 2008924657

British Library Cataloguing in Publication data

A catalogue record for this book is available from the British Library

ISBN 978-1-84787-511-2
ISBN 978-1-84787-512-9 (pbk)

Typeset by C&M Digitals (P) Ltd., Chennai, India
Printed and bound by CPI Group (UK) Ltd, Croydon, CR0 4YY
Printed on paper from sustainable resources

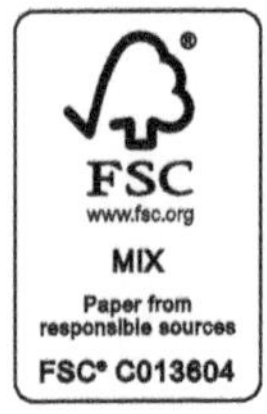

Contents

Acknowledgements

Every effort has been made to trace all the copyright holders, but if any have been inadvertently overlooked the publishers will be pleased to make the necessary arrangement at the first opportunity.

Pieces 1–4
Reproduced courtesy of St Christopher's Hospice, Sydenham, Kent.

Piece 5
A woman and a boy visiting a man in hospital, Kathe Kollwitz, © DACS 2008, image supplied courtesy of Wellcome Library, London.

Piece 6
A deathbed scene, Alfred Kubin, © Eberhard Spangenberg/(DACS, 2008), image supplied courtesy of Wellcome Library, London.

Piece 7
© Margareta Kern 2006, 2007. Reproduced by kind permission of Margareta Kern.

Piece 8
Reproduced courtesy of Ann Brodie.

Piece 9
The death of Chatterton, Henry Wallis 1856, copyright © Tate, London 2008. Reproduced with permission.

Piece 10
R. Schäfer, 1989 *Dead Faces* in Granta (Death), 27, Summer, pp. 193–210.

Piece 11
The dissection of a beautiful young woman, J.H. Hasselhorst, courtesy of Wellcome Library, London.

Piece 12
Human bones in Paris catacombs, istock image 4487773, Phillip Jones Photography.

Piece 13
Mass grave, Belsen, Hulton Archive/Getty Images. Reproduced with permission.

Pieces 14 and 15
© Joe Earle

Piece 16
© Caroline Bartholomew

Piece 17
© 2004 Bob Bednar. Reproduced with permission.

Piece 18
Memorial Quilt, Scotland, 2004, originated by Gilly Thomson and Ruby Henderson. Courtesy of The Compassionate Friends (TCF), an organisation of bereaved parents and their families (www.tcf.org.uk/)

Piece 20
Excerpts from *Vicky Angel*, by Jacqueline Wilson, Corgi, 2000. Reproduced by permission of David Higham Associates Ltd.

Piece 21
'Do Not Go Gentle Into That Good Night', from *The Collected Poems*, New Directions, 1952. Reprinted by permission of David Higham Associates on behalf of the author.

'Do Not Go Gentle Into That Good Night' by Dylan Thomas, from *The Poems of Dylan Thomas*, copyright © 1952 by Dylan Thomas. Reprinted by permission of New Directions Publishing Corp.

Piece 22
'Ode to a nightingale' [final three verses] by John Keats, p.190, Dent & Sons Ltd.

Piece 23
'Funeral Blues' by Wystan Hugh Auden, from *Collected Poems*, ed. Edward Mendelson, Faber and Faber Ltd, 1991, © the Estate of Wystan Hugh Auden. Reprinted with permission.

'Funeral Blues', copyright 1940 and renewed 1968 by W.H. Auden, from *Collected Poems* by W.H. Auden. Used by permission of Random House, Inc.

Piece 25
Wilfred Owen, 'Anthem for doomed youth', from John Stallworthy, ed., *Wilfred Owen: The War Poems* (London: Chatto & Windus, 1994). Reprinted with permission.

Piece 26
'Aftermath', from Collected Poems of Siegfried Sassoon by Siegfried Sassoon, copyright 1918, 1920 by E.P. Dutton. Copyright 1936, 1946, 1947, 1948 by Siegfried Sassoon. Used by permission of Viking Penguin, a division of Penguin Group (USA) Inc.

'Aftermath', Collected Poems 1908–1956 by Siegfried Sassoon. Copyright © Siegfried Sassoon by kind permission of the Estate of George Sassoon.

Piece 32
'Obituary – Dame Cicely Saunders', July 15, 2005, *The Times*. Copyright © *The Times*. Reprinted with permission.

Piece 33
Pamela Roberts, 'Here Today and Cyberspace Tomorrow: Memorials and Bereavement Support on the Web', reprinted with permission from *Generations*, Summer 2005, pp. 41–6. Copyright © 2005 American Society on Aging, San Francisco, California. www.asaging.org.

Piece 34
Excerpts from Winston's Wish: For young people http://winstonswish.org.uk/foryoungpeople/say/ reproduced with permission.

Piece 35
Excerpts from Bereavement UK: The garden of tranquillity http://bereavementuk.co.uk/tranqui.htm reproduced with permission.

Piece 36
Text excerpts and images from Andrea Rouen's farewell http://ousasw.org.uk/andrea.html reproduced by kind permission of Roz Evans, Kate Graham, Diana Isserlis. 'The Dash' © Linda Ellis 1996 (www.lindaellis.net).

Piece 37
Excerpts from 'Cancergiggles' by Cass Brown www.cancergiggles.blog-city.com/live_with_cancer_1.htm reproduced by kind permission of Kim Brown.

Piece 39
Katja Becker and Martin H. Schmidt, 'When kids seek help on-line: Internet chat rooms and suicide', *Reclaiming Children and Youth*, 13(4), Winter, pp. 229–30. Originally published as a letter to the editor in *Journal of American Academy of Child and Adolescent Psychiatry*, March 2004 issue (43: 3: pp. 245–7). Reprinted by permission of Lippincott Williams & Wilkins.

Piece 43
Excerpts from *Precious Lives* by Margaret Forster, published by Chatto & Windus. Reprinted by permission of The Random House Group Ltd and The Sayle Literary Agency.

Piece 44
Elizabeth Young, Clive Seale and Michael Bury, 'It's not like family going, is it? Negotiating friendship boundaries towards the end of life', *Mortality*, 3(1), 1998, Taylor & Francis Ltd, reprinted with the permission of the publisher (Taylor & Francis Ltd, www.informaworld.com).

Piece 47
Cynda Hylton-Rushton, 'Caregiver suffering is a dimension of end-of-life care', reprinted with permission from *The American Nurse*, November/December 2001, published by the American Nurses Association.

Piece 48
Excerpt from 'On Fighting' from *BETTER: a Surgeon's Notes on Performance* by Atul Gawande. Copyright © 2007 by Atul Gawande. Reprinted by permission of Henry Holt and Company, LLC and Profile Books.

Piece 49
Nancy A. Hodgson, Sheila Segal, Maria Weidinger, and Mary Beth Linde, 'Being there: Contributions of the nurse, social worker and chaplain during and after a death', reprinted with permission from *Generations*, Summer 2004, 28(2): pp. 47–52. Copyright © 2004 American Society on Aging, San Francisco, California. www.asaging.org.

Piece 55
'A Grief Observed' by C.S. Lewis copyright © C.S. Lewis Pte. Ltd 1961. Extract reprinted by permission.

Piece 66
Stuart Todd, 'Silenced endings: Death, dying and learning disabilities', a summary report of a research study funded by the Henry Smith Charity, Welsh Centre for Learning Disabilities, Cardiff

University. Reproduced by kind permission of the author.

Piece 68
Prathap Tharyan, 'Traumatic bereavement and the Asian Tsunami: Perspectives from Tamil Nadu, India', extract taken with permission from an article originally published in *Bereavement Care* 2005; 24(2): 21–4. © Cruse Bereavement Care, PO Box 800, Richmond TW9 1RG, UK.

Piece 69
Lesley Moreland, 'Ruth: Death by murder', in Dickenson, Johnson, Samson Katz (eds), *Death, Dying and Bereavement*, 2nd edn. SAGE, 2000, pp. 376–8. Reproduced by kind permission of the publisher and author.

Piece 71
'When Disaster Strikes: Reflections on personal experience of disaster', www.disasteraction.org.uk/support/da_guide08.pdf, DisasterAction. Reproduced by kind permission of DisasterAction. Survivors and bereaved people from UK and overseas disasters founded DisasterAction (DA) in 1991, as an independent, British-based charity. An advocacy and advisory service, their purpose is to raise awareness of the needs of those directly affected by disaster and to offer support to survivors and bereaved. www.disasteraction.org.uk

Piece 72
Tom Heller, 'Personal and medical memories from Hillsborough', in Dickenson, Johnson, Samson Katz (eds), *Death, Dying and Bereavement*, 2nd edn. SAGE, 2000, pp. 371–5. Originally published in BMJ, vol. 299, 1989, pp. 1596–8. Reproduced by permission of *BMJ*.

Piece 76
Excerpts from 'Hospital ghosts and hauntings', Paranormal Database (www.paranormaldatabase.com/reports/hospital.php). Reproduced by kind permission of Darren Mann.

Piece 79
Extract from *The Traveller-Gypsies*, Judith Okely 1983, Copyright © Cambridge University Press, reproduced with permission.

Piece 80
From 'If the Spirit Moves You' by Justine Picardie, copyright © 2001 by Justine Picardie. Used by permission of Riverhead Books, an imprint of Penguin Group (USA) Inc.

Extract from 'If the Spirit Moves You' by Justine Picardie, Pan Macmillan, 2001. Copyright © Justine Picardie 2001. Reprinted with permission.

Piece 83
Roger Dobson, 'Sparkling epitaphs: From jewels to web portraits, we've moved on from the tombstone', *The Times*, September 10th, www.timesonline.co.uk/tol/life_and_style/health/features/article564339.ece. Copyright © Roger Dobson/NI Syndication. Reprinted with permission.

Making Sense of Death, Dying and Bereavement: An Introduction

Sarah Earle, Caroline Bartholomew and Carol Komaromy

This anthology has been developed as a sourcebook and designed to stimulate reflection on the different ways in which death, dying and bereavement can be understood. The book is organised into seven parts, each exploring a distinct theme. Whilst each part can be read in turn, they can also be read independently, or you may wish to dip in and out of the pieces which most interest you. Most importantly, by drawing on a unique collection of personal accounts – many of which have been specially written for this volume – this anthology offers an insight into the feelings and experiences of those who are affected by death, dying and bereavement.

Part I: Visual Images of Death, Dying and Disposal offers a selection of images which represent both traditional and more contemporary representations of death and dying. For example, here you can find images of graves and post-mortem photography. Also included is a death certificate, images of roadside memorials from the United States, England and elsewhere in Europe, and examples of artwork created by hospice service users.

Visual representations of death and dying are evocative but the subject of death, dying and bereavement is also richly represented in literature. Part II: Death and Dying in Poetry, Fiction and the Media offers a selection of both newly commissioned and previously published poetry, including poetry from World War I. A selection of edited extracts from classic and contemporary literature, including children's fiction, can also be found. An obituary of Cicely Saunders is also included in this part of the book.

In Part III: Death, Dying and Bereavement on the World Wide Web, attention turns to the role of the World Wide Web and its transformative potential in the field of death, dying and bereavement. The widespread availability and accessibility of the Web has meant that it is increasingly used by those who are dying or have been bereaved, as well as by those who want to find out more about these issues. Part III focuses on the role of the Web in the provision of bereavement information, memorialisation, and as a forum for community support and communication.

Part IV: Caring for People at the End of Life draws on the personal accounts of friends and family members to explore the experiences of those caring for someone who is dying. The contributions explore the rewards, challenges and regrets, as well as some of the ethical dilemmas. This part of the book also includes contributions from people who provide care at the end of life in a professional capacity. Here, you can find contributions from nurses, doctors, hospice support workers and hospital porters, amongst others.

In the next part of the book, attention turns to the feelings and experiences of those who have been bereaved, and considers the important role of professional care-givers. Part V: When Someone Dies includes a diversity of contributions, but the selection of pieces give consideration to expected as well as sudden and unexpected deaths.

The experiences of people who survive or who have been bereaved following traumatic death, mass death and disaster are unique, and so Part VI: Reflecting on Traumatic Death, Mass Death and Disaster focuses specifically on these. This part of the book includes contributions from a forensic ecologist and a crisis management consultant, as well as the account of someone charged with the responsibility for returning personal property following mass death and disaster. Whilst recognising that the experiences of people who survive disasters are diverse, Part VI draws on personal accounts of those affected by (amongst others) the disaster at the football stadium in Hillsborough, the Asian Tsunami, and the terrorist attacks on the World Trade Centre in New York.

The final part of this book focuses on a much debated and disputed question: what happens after death? In Part VII: Making Sense of the After-life and Life After Death, personal accounts of apparitions and the stories of those who seek to communicate with those who have died are presented. These contributions offer different ways of making sense of the after-life and of the experiences of those who are bereaved. Part VII also explores life after death and ways of commemorating and memorialising the lives of people who have died.

Part I

Visual Images of Death, Dying and Disposal

Introduction

Sarah Earle and Carol Komaromy

Death is universal and concerns everybody, but the way it is understood changes across time and space. Ideas about death can be expressed in different ways, and some of these different forms of expression can be seen in the collection of pieces within this anthology. Part I begins by offering a selection of visual images of death, dying and disposal. These images range from representations of death and dying in fine art to (amongst others) documentary and more contemporary photography.

Visual representations of death, dying and disposal can be challenging, as well as evocative. For example, death can be represented in the news media as something shocking or sensational; in literature as something dramatic or romantic; in films as tragic or violent; and, in art, all of these meanings can be found.

Some of the images presented here have been reproduced with kind permission, whereas others are printed for the first time. The viewer is left to engage with, and interpret, the images, some of which will inevitably resonate with personal meanings. It is this mixture of private emotions and public image that makes representations both powerfully symbolic and emotionally stirring. More than this, however, the images of death and dying in contemporary society both reflect and shape the relationship that its citizens have with death and dying.

1
Afghanistan Woman

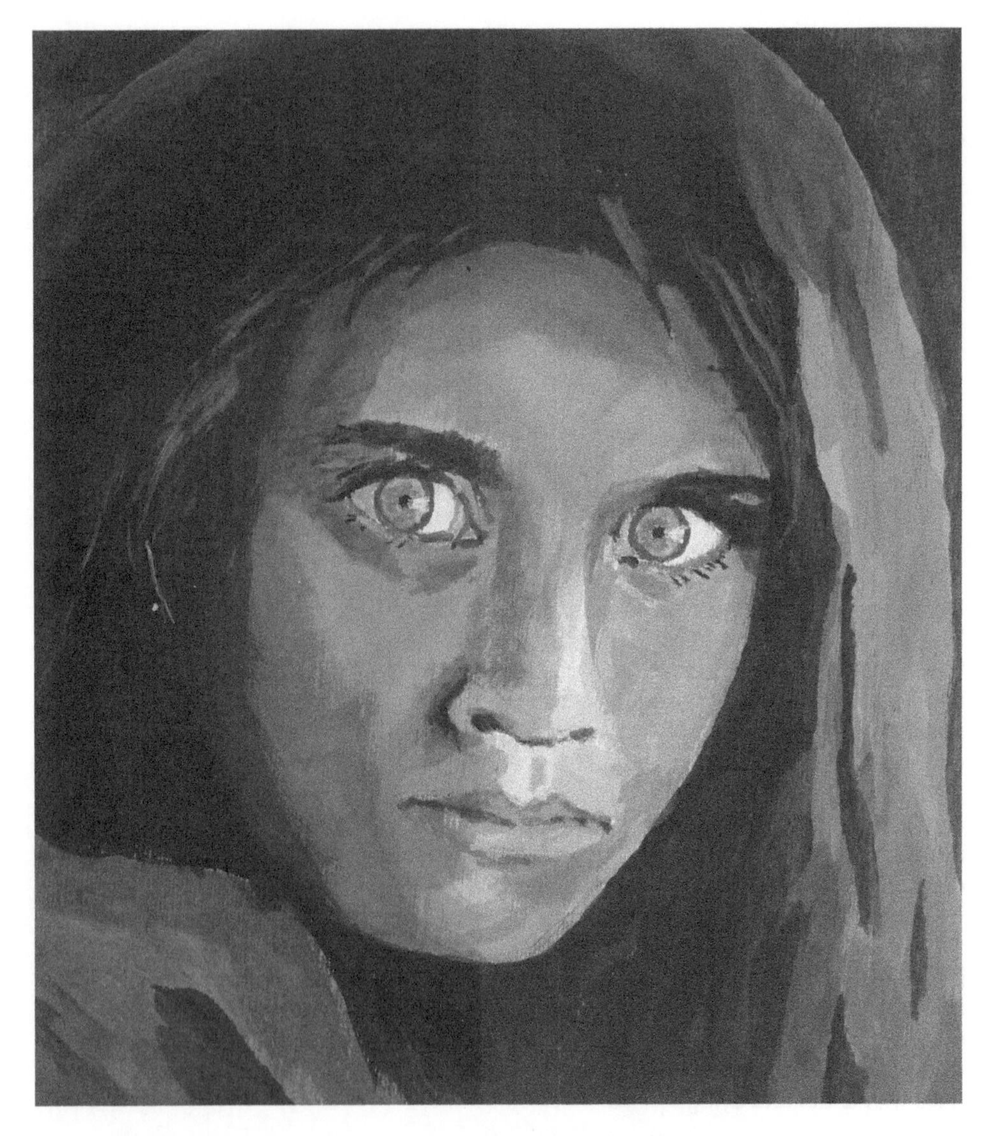

A painting created as part of an 'Arts for Life' project, enabling people coming to the end of life to tell their story. Courtesy of St Christopher's Hospice, Sydenham, Kent.

2
Sunrise

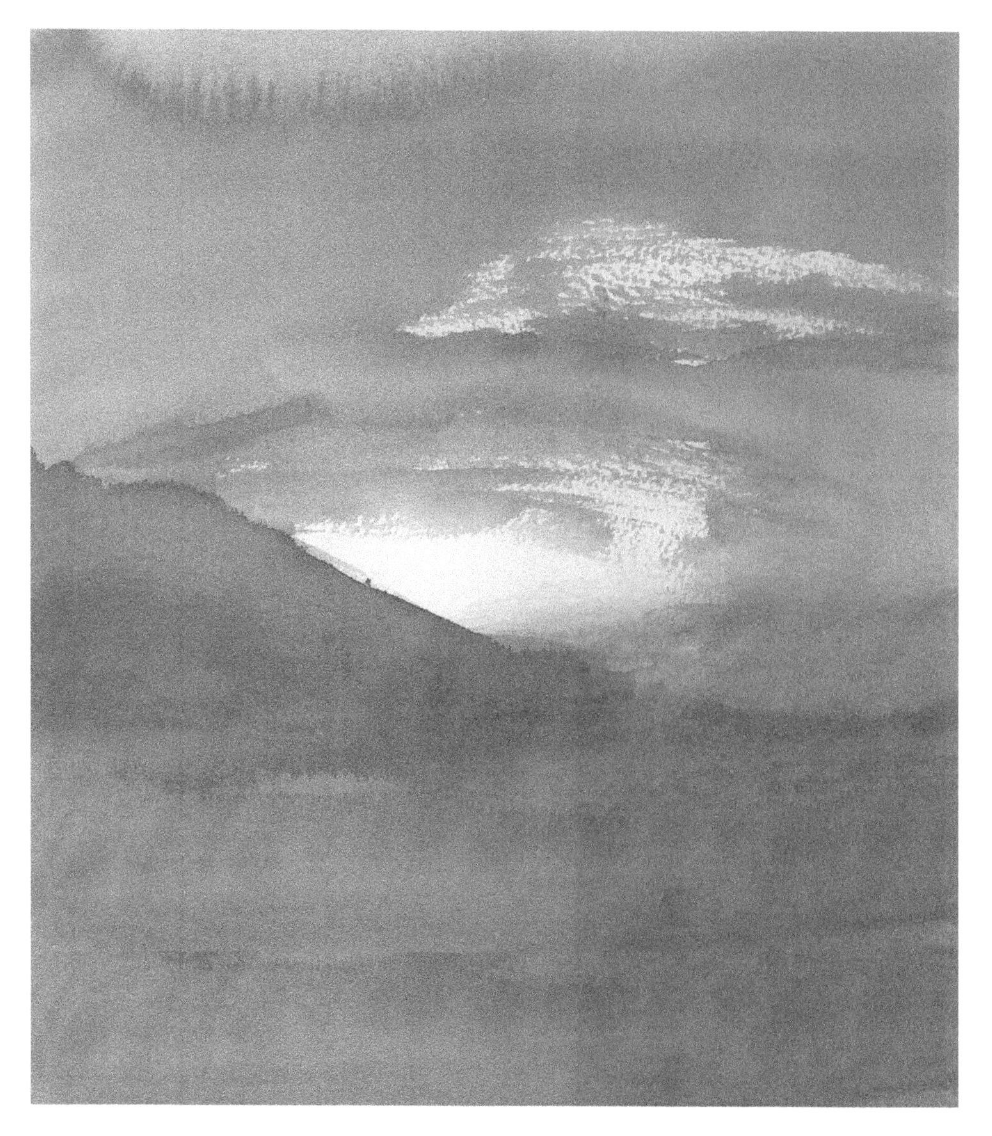

A painting created as part of an 'Arts for Life' project, enabling people coming to the end of life to tell their story. Courtesy of St Christopher's Hospice.

3
Purple Planet

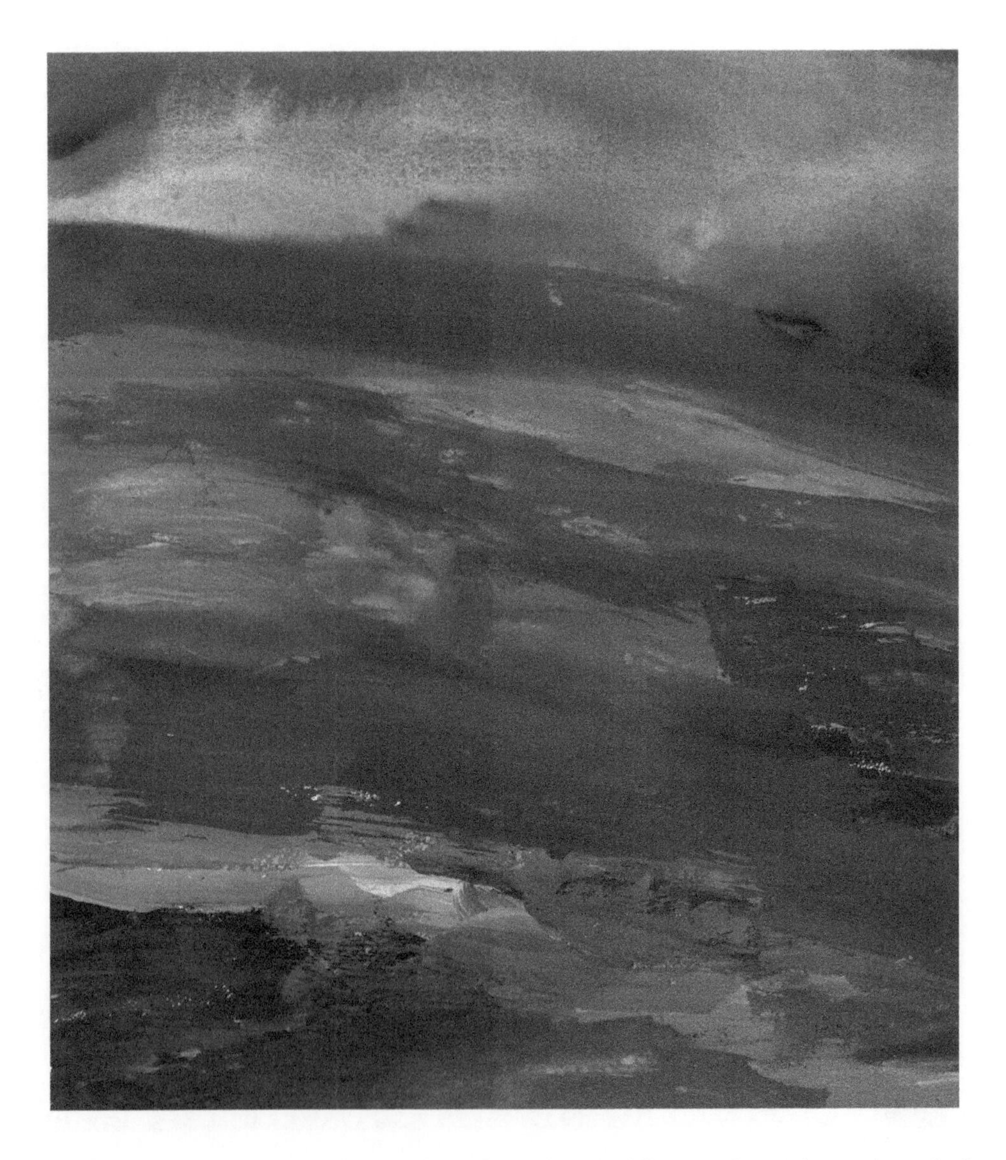

A painting created as part of an 'Arts for Life' project, enabling people coming to the end of life to tell their story. Courtesy of St Christopher's Hospice.

4
Mask

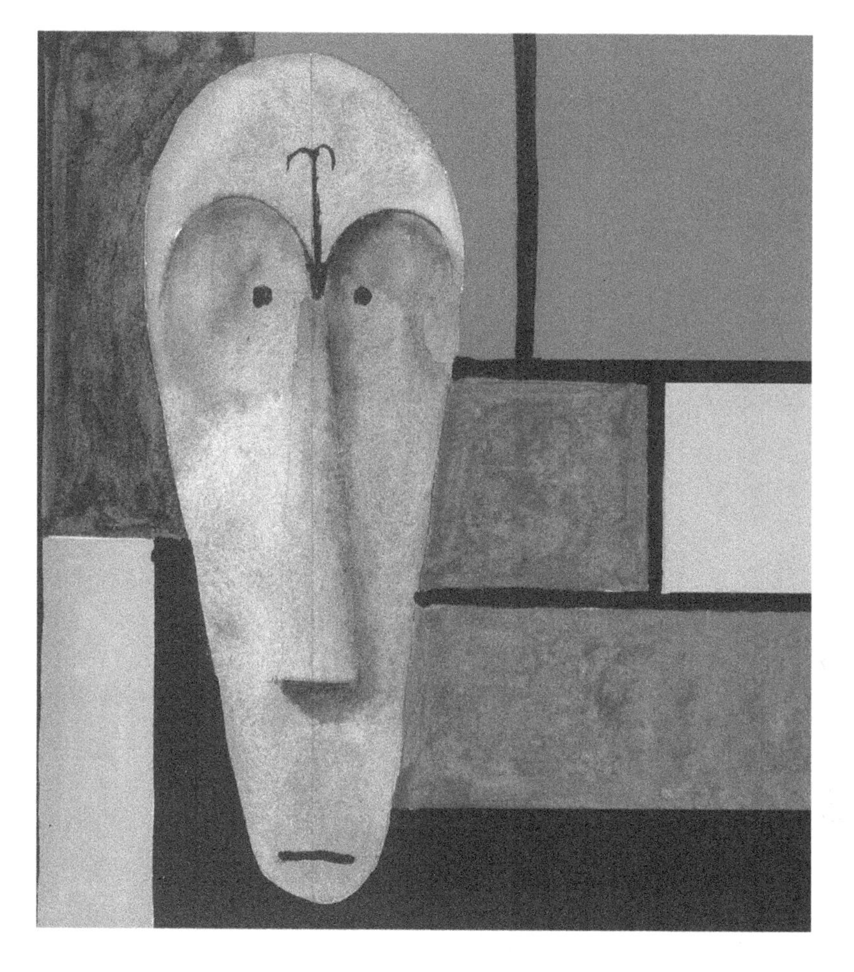

A painting created as part of an 'Arts for Life' project, enabling people coming to the end of life to tell their story. Courtesy of St Christopher's Hospice.

5
A Woman and a Boy Visiting a Man in Hospital, Woodcut by Käthe Kollwitz

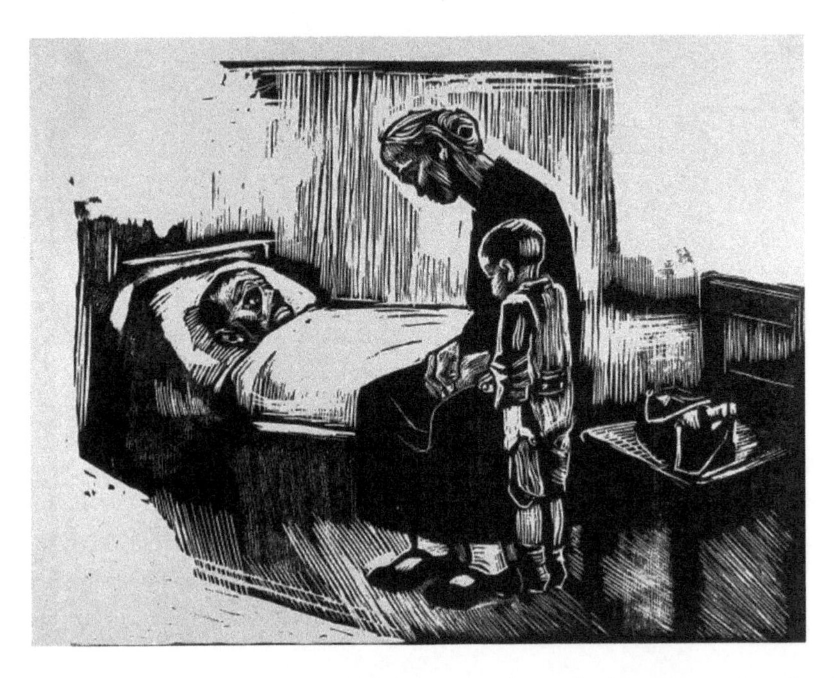

Throughout the twentieth century, hospitals became an increasingly common place for death. Kollwitz's woodcut reflects this trend as well as the nineteenth-century artistic use of 'death art' to explore family relationships.

A woman and a boy visiting a man in hospital, Kathe Kollwitz, © DACS 2008, image supplied courtesy of Wellcome Library, London.

6
A Deathbed Scene, Etching by Alfred Kubin

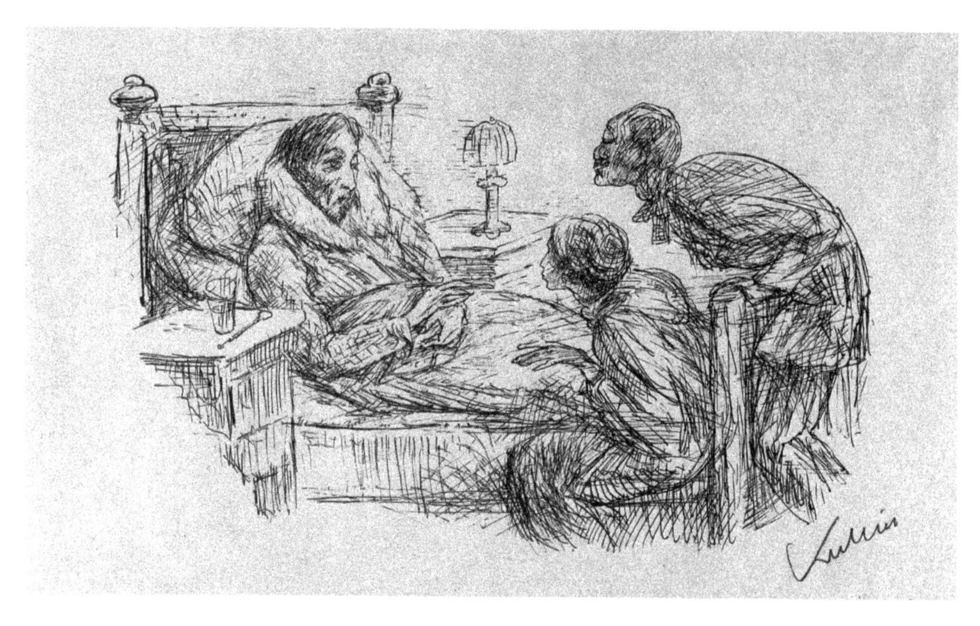

The nineteenth century witnessed a shift in social trends from the custom of visiting the dying to that of viewing the person after death, with the former being reserved predominantly for close family.

A deathbed scene, Alfred Kubin, © Eberhard Spangenberg/(DACS, 2008), image supplied courtesy of Wellcome Library, London.

7
Margareta Kern: Clothes for Death

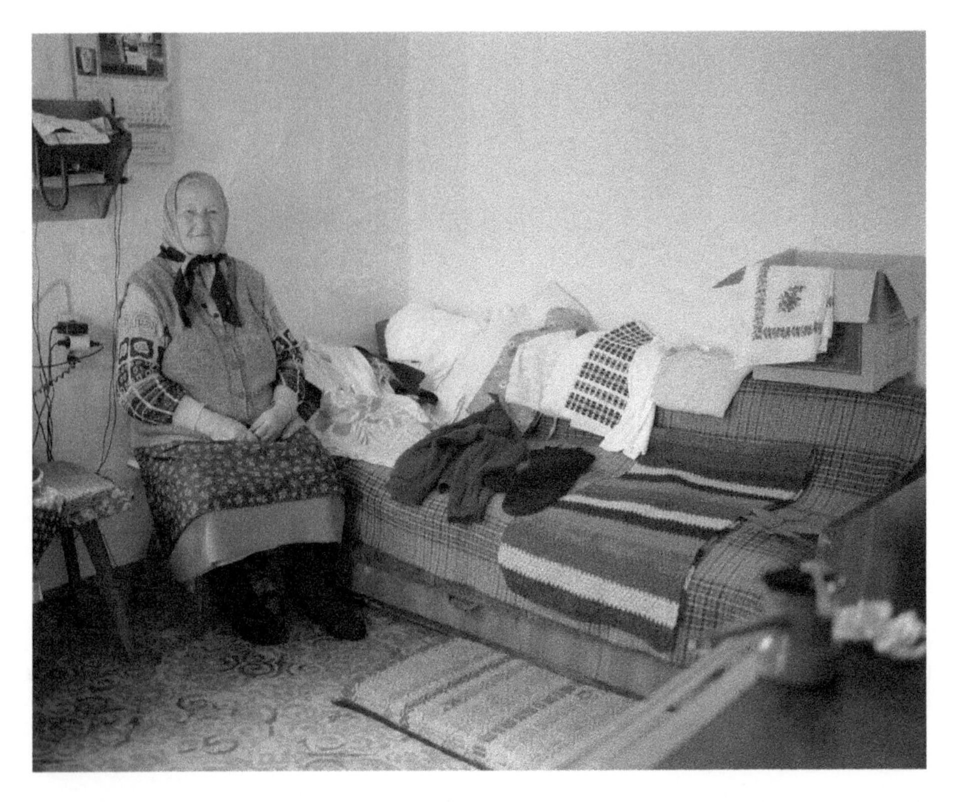

Mila (Banjica, Bosnia and Herzegovina), 2007, from the Clothes for Death series of photographs.

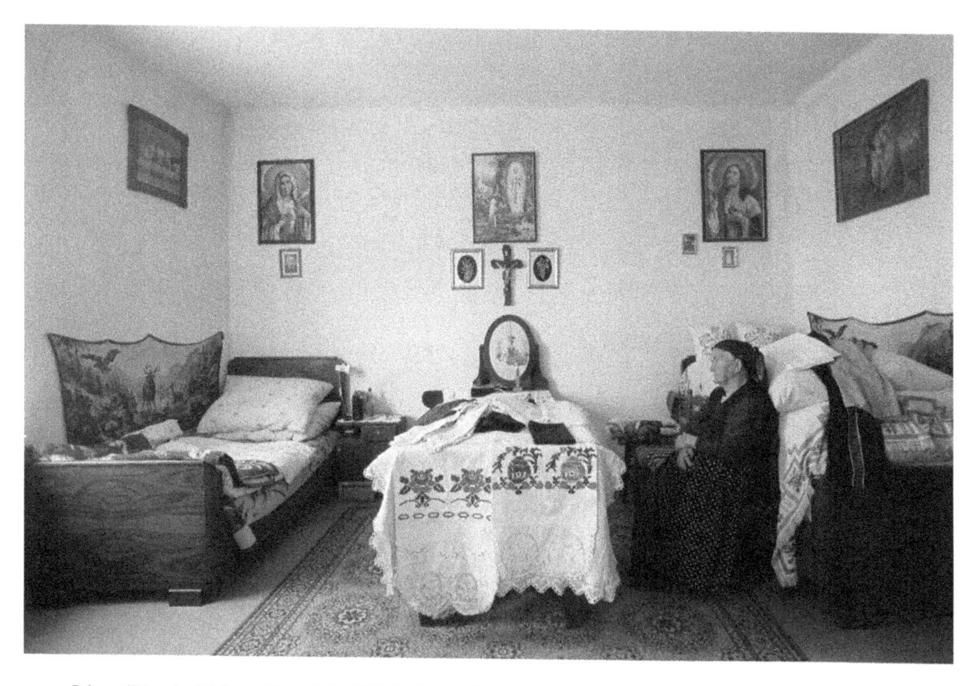

Liza (Donja Vrba, Croatia), 2006, from the Clothes for Death series of photographs.

Margareta Kern: Clothes for Death*

Clothes for Death (Odjeca za Smrt) is a research-based art project documenting women in Croatia and Bosnia & Herzegovina who prepare the clothes in which they wish to be buried (see plates on pp. 10 and 11). I started the project with an initial journey in Autumn 2006, and my current journey started on the 15 March 2007. The project is funded by Arts Council England.

Saturday, 31 Mar 2007

I always leave to the women to arrange how they want to present the clothes; it is their personal choice how they spread it out and nearly everyone immediately has their own notion of how they like it to be arranged for photographing.

Tuesday, 3 Apr 2007

I am struck by the way women keep their pieces of clothing: wrapped in a sheet, or in travel bags, plastic bags, suitcases … One of the women, Jovana, who is 97 years old, pulled out a dusty old suitcase from underneath the bed and inside it was a floral dress, long woollen socks (which she probably knitted), petticoat and many family photographs. It was as though she was preparing for a journey and needed to be ready at any moment …

The Orthodox priest told me that in his view, the custom of preparing clothes for death (or funeral, as some also say) comes from the tradition of preparing one's best suit or a dress for the Sunday mass and preparing for the meeting with God. A person needed to be ready and in 'Sunday's best' when meeting God …

This stayed with me and I think he has definitely touched on some of the religious background to this still mysterious custom. It has also made me think about the connection between fashion and religion …

*This is an edited extract of Margareta Kern's blog on www.a-n.co.uk/projects_unedited

8
A Death Certificate

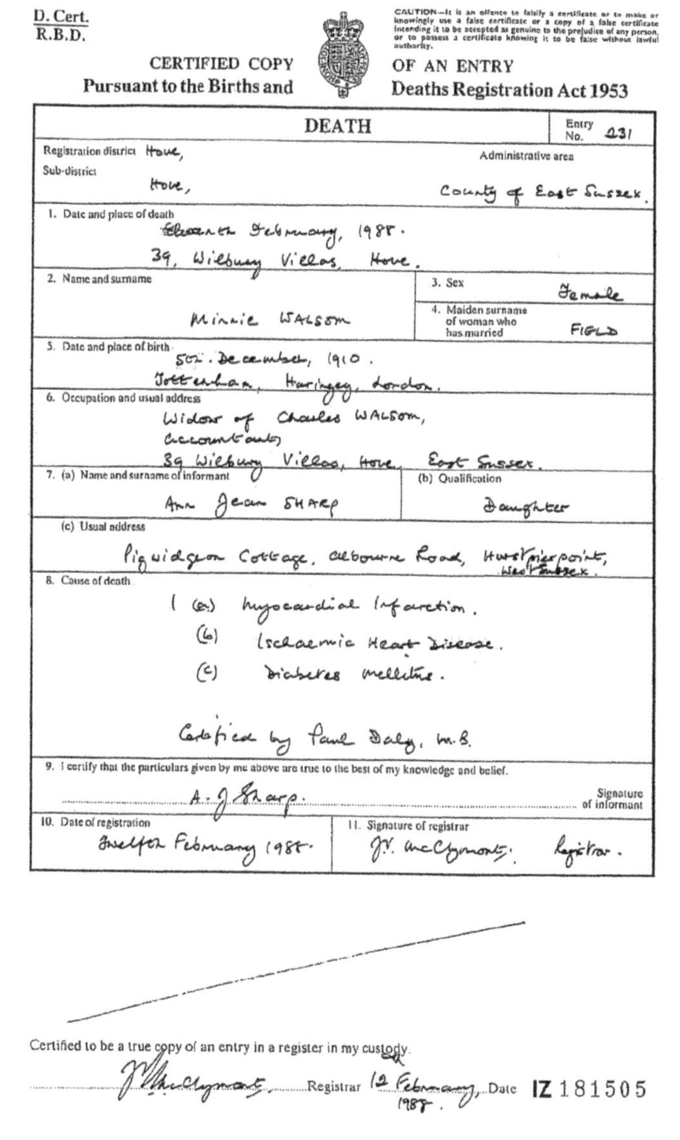

D. Cert.
R.B.D.

CAUTION—It is an offence to falsify a certificate or to make or knowingly use a false certificate or a copy of a false certificate intending it to be accepted as genuine to the prejudice of any person, or to possess a certificate knowing it to be false without lawful authority.

CERTIFIED COPY OF AN ENTRY
Pursuant to the Births and Deaths Registration Act 1953

DEATH — Entry No. 231

Registration district Hove, — Administrative area
Sub-district Hove, — County of East Sussex.

1. Date and place of death
Eleventh February, 1988.
39, Wilbury Villas, Hove.

2. Name and surname
Minnie WALSOM

3. Sex
Female

4. Maiden surname of woman who has married
FIELD

5. Date and place of birth
5th. December, 1910.
Tottenham, Haringey, London.

6. Occupation and usual address
Widow of Charles WALSOM,
Accountant,
39 Wilbury Villas, Hove, East Sussex.

7. (a) Name and surname of informant
Ann Jean SHARP

(b) Qualification
Daughter

(c) Usual address
Pigwidgeon Cottage, Albourne Road, Hurstpierpoint, West Sussex.

8. Cause of death
I (a) Myocardial Infarction.
(b) Ischaemic Heart Disease.
(c) Diabetes Mellitus.

Certified by Paul Daly, M.B.

9. I certify that the particulars given by me above are true to the best of my knowledge and belief.
A. J. Sharp. — Signature of informant

10. Date of registration
Twelfth February 1988.

11. Signature of registrar
J.V. McClymont. Registrar.

Certified to be a true copy of an entry in a register in my custody.
J. McClymont ....Registrar 12 February 1988 ....Date IZ 181505

Certificate of death for Minnie Walsom who died on 11 February 1988. Courtesy of Ann Brodie.

9
The Death of Chatterton

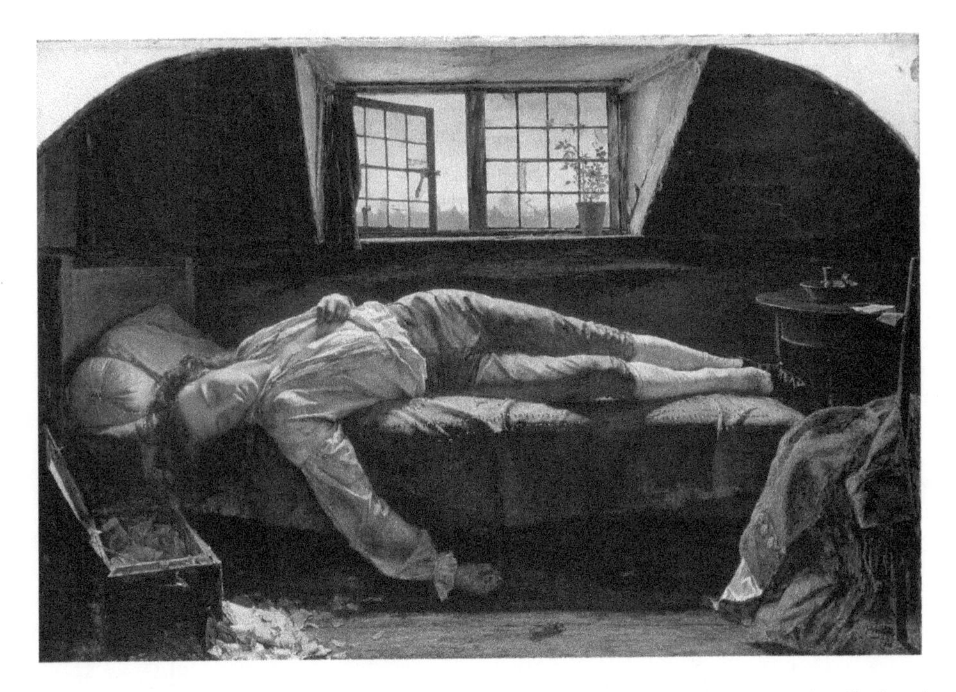

A painting by Henry Wallis of the Romantic English poet Thomas Chatterton, who died at the age of 17.

10
Dead Faces of a Girl and a Man

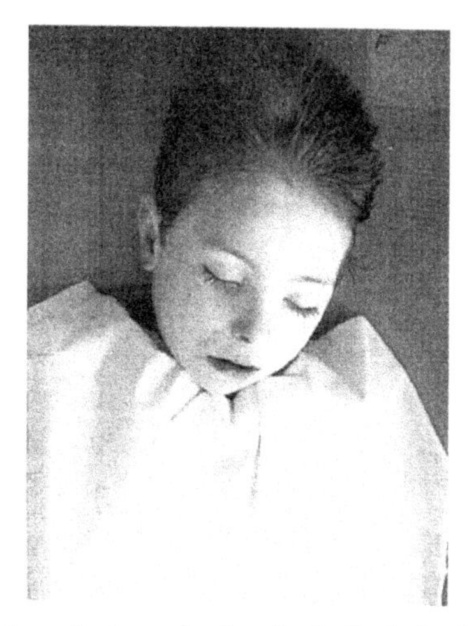

Dead face of a girl, a post-mortem photograph taken in the Pathological Institute of Charité, Berlin.

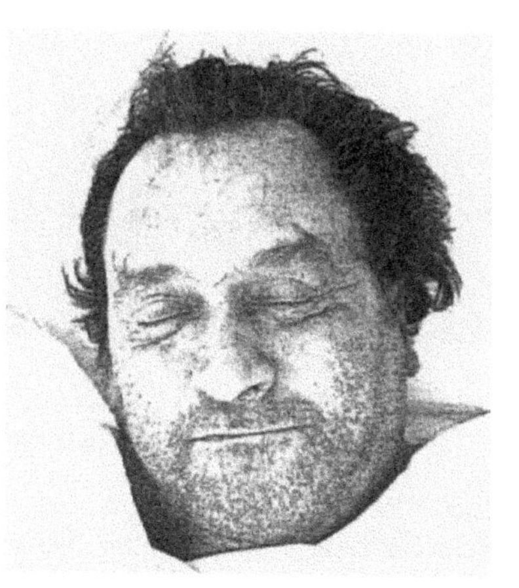

Dead face of a man, a post-mortem photograph taken in the Pathological Institute of Charité, Berlin.

R. Schäfer, 1989 *Dead Faces* in Granta (Death), 27, Summer, pp.193–210.

11
The Dissection of a Beautiful Young Woman

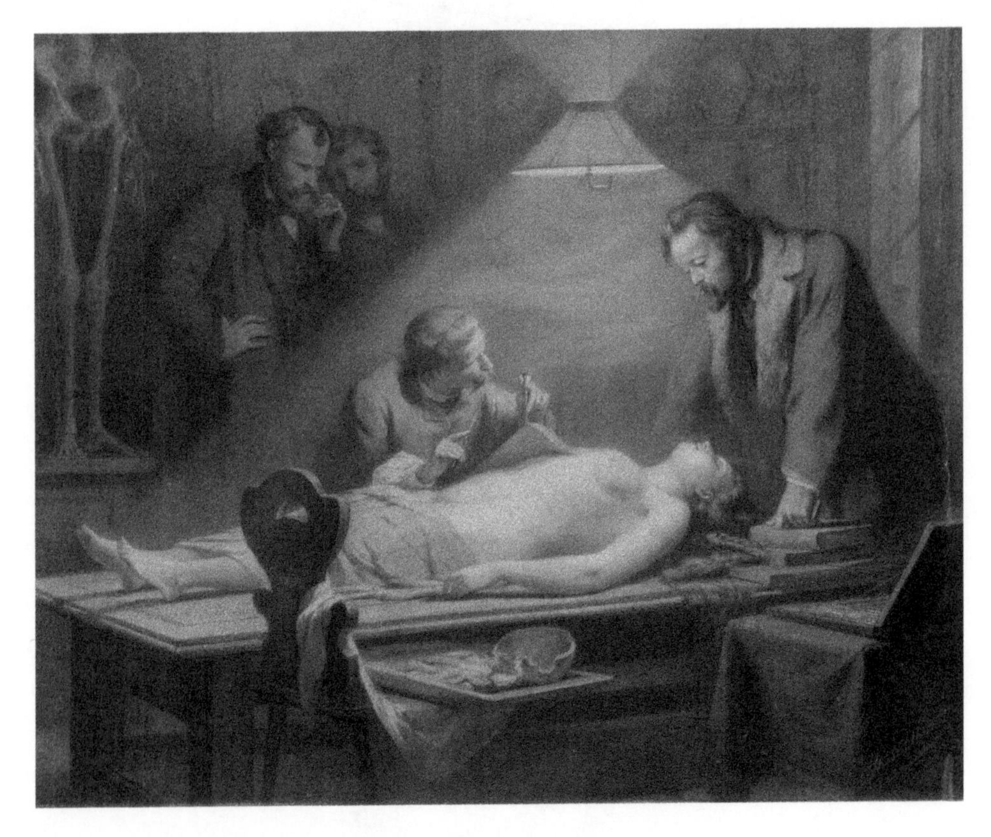

The dissection of a beautiful young woman directed by J.Ch.G. Lucae (1814–1885), chalk drawing by J.H. Hasselhorst, 1864

The drawing depicts the dissection of an 18-year-old suicide victim, selected for her 'attractive proportions'. The object of the dissection was to determine the 'ideal proportions' of the female body. During the nineteenth century, yound dead bodies were celebrated as objects of desire (see also A. Davidsson Bremborg in Part III, pp. 76–9).

The dissection of a beautiful young woman, J.H. Hasselhorst, courtesy of Wellcome Library, London.

12
Human Bones in Paris Catacombs

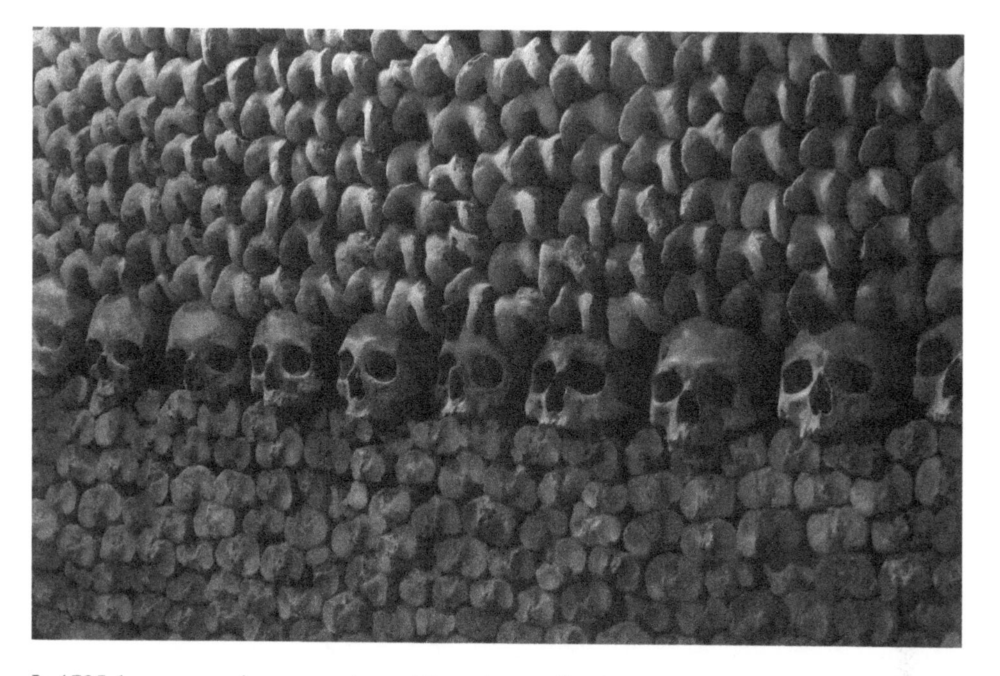

In 1785, human remains were exhumed from the overflowing cemeteries in Paris and the bones relocated in the tunnels of disused quarries. Parts of the catacombs are open to the public.

Human bones in Paris catacombs, istock image 4487773, Phillip Jones Photography.

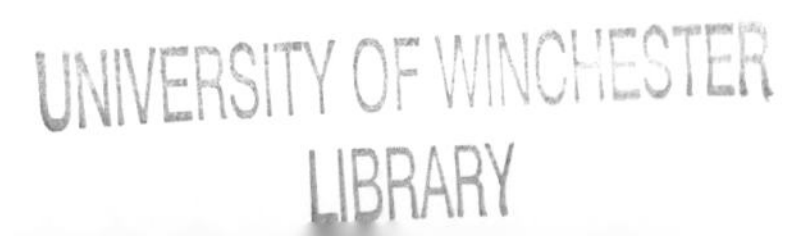

13
Mass Grave, Belsen

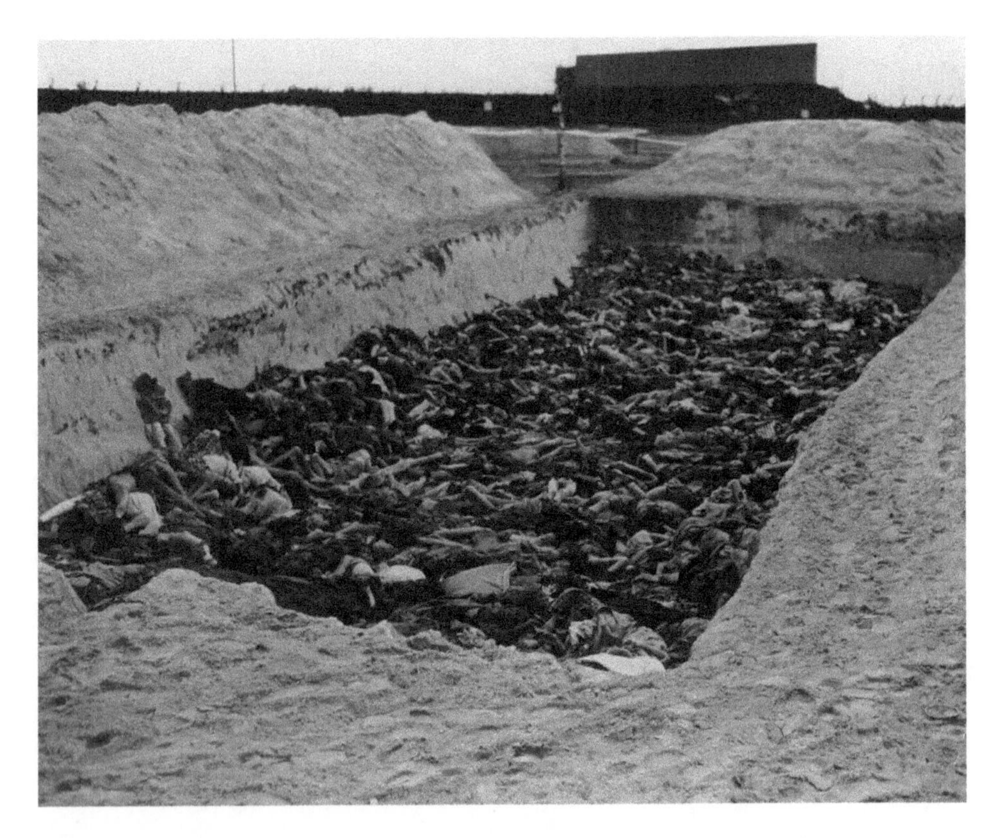

April 1945: View of emaciated bodies heaped on top of one another in one of the mass graves at the Belsen concentration camp, after the camp was liberated during the advance of the British 2nd Army in World War II, Belsen, Germany (see also C. Komaromy in Part VI, pp. 169–70).

14
Abandoned Grave

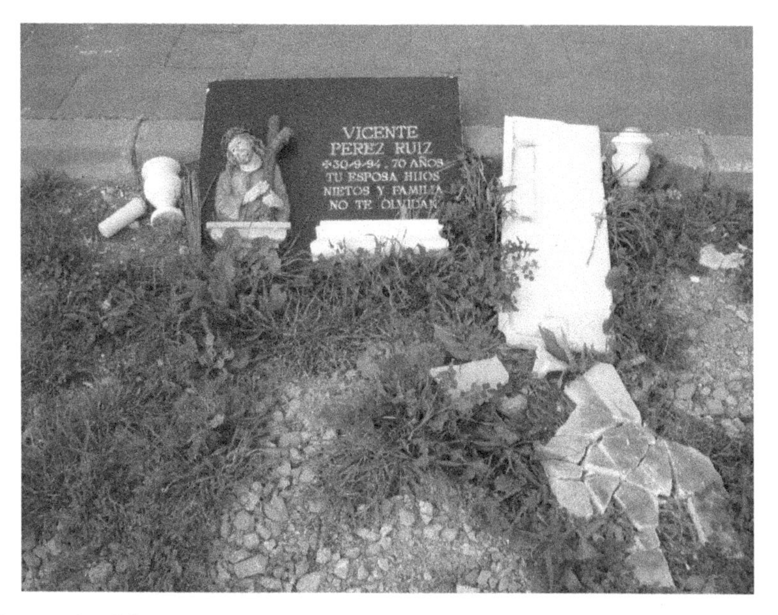

Inscription reads: 'Vincente Perez Ruiz, 30 September 1994, 70 years, your wife, children, grandchildren and family will not forget you', Cementerio de San José, La Línea de la Concepción, Spain.

15
Roadside Memorial, Avenida España, Cadiz, Spain

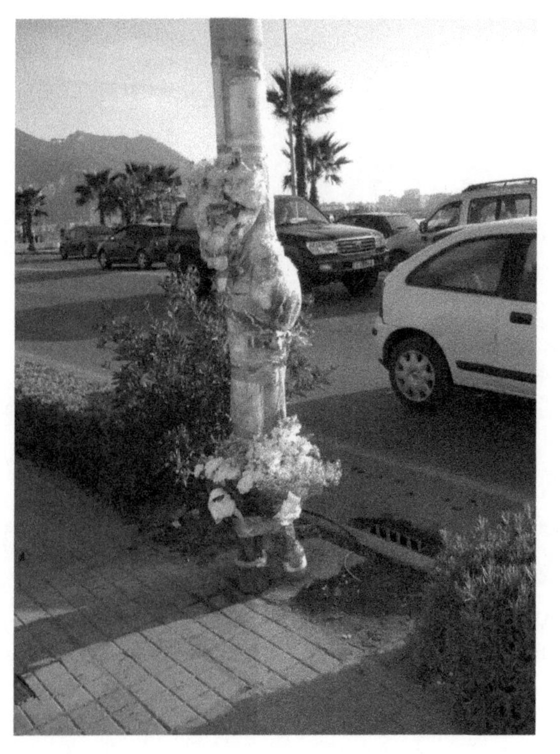

Roadside memorial commemorates the life of a young woman.

16
Roadside Memorial, Groveway, Milton Keynes, UK

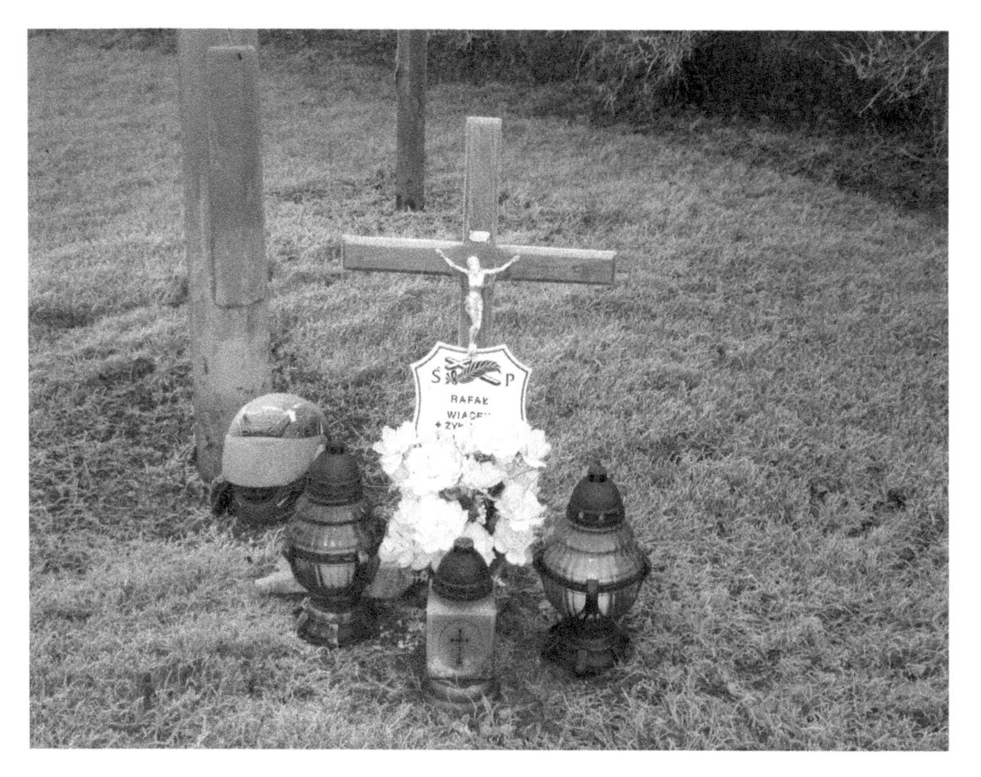

Memorial to a motorcyclist killed at a road junction.

17
Roadside Memorials and the Public Health

PLEASE
DON'T
DRINK
AND
DRIVE
IN MEMORY OF
BARBARA HOWELL

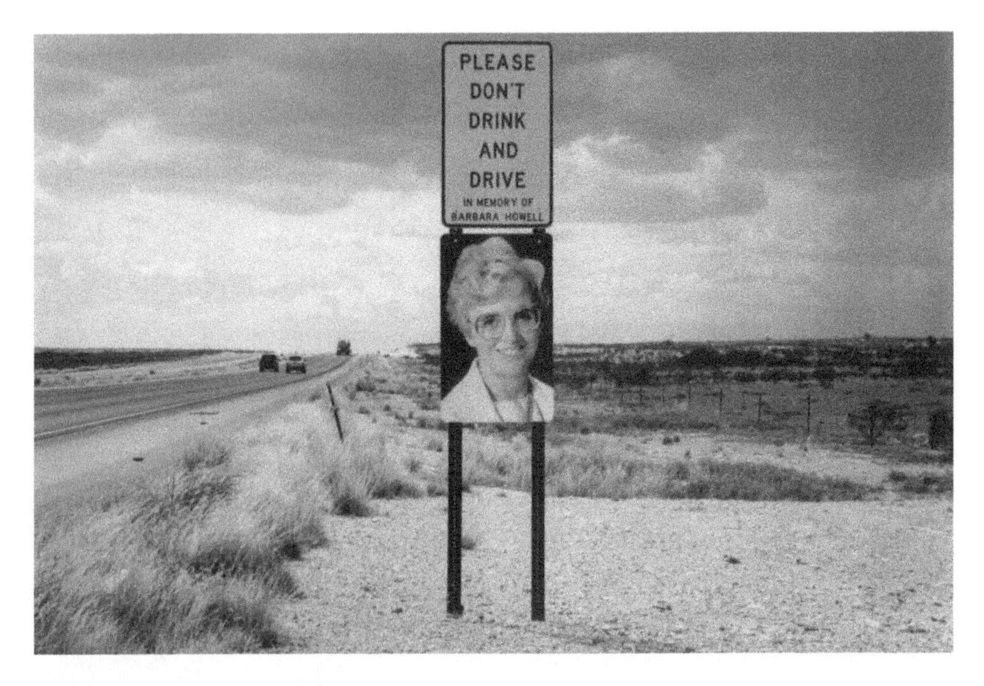

In New Mexico the state has embraced the practice of roadside memorialisation, using it in official drink-driving messages.

Making space on the side of the road

The first few times I stopped at memorials, I felt horribly self-conscious, almost shameful. If you have ever stopped at a stranger's memorial, you'll know what I mean. If you haven't, I hope some day you will. You feel as though you have been suddenly transported into a stranger's bedroom, and there are people watching you look through other people's stuff. There I am on the side of the road looking at, photographing, and sometimes touching the intimately symbolic objects of a person's life, and I don't know who they are or how they lived or how they died.

Any yet, these are not bedrooms, or even living rooms, but spaces on the side of the road visible to all who drive by.

Whatever else we might see communicated by the memorials, one thing rings through clearly: that the people who attach crosses and flowers to fences and trees and guardrails and build grottoes and shrines along the right of way think that they have the right to do so – think that there is room for them (or at least *should* be room for them) in public space. In some states – Texas, for instance – it is illegal to construct and maintain a roadside memorial, but in New Mexico the state has embraced the practice, using it in billboards and other official public media DWI [driving whilst intoxicated] messages (see also A. Árnarson, Part V, pp. 150–1).

18
Memorial Quilt, Scotland 2004

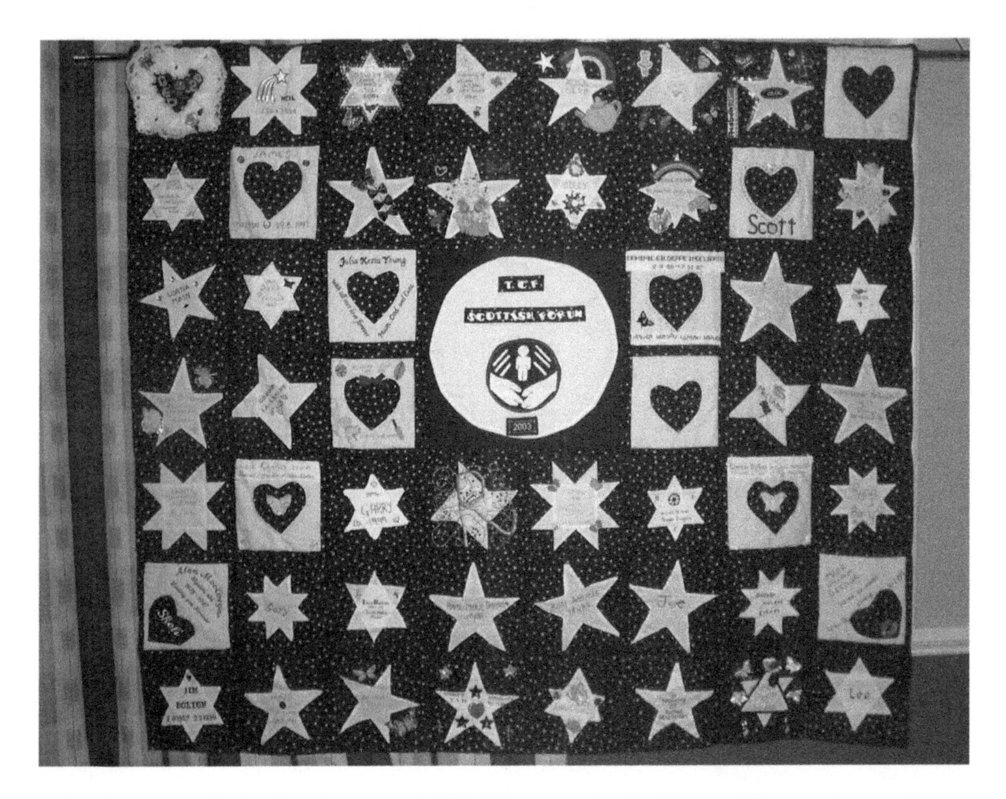

A few years ago, Ruby Henderson and Gilly Thomson decided it would be good to produce a Scottish TCF quilt which was different from the 'butterfly' quilts of the UK. Inspiration came from the Eskimo legend of the stars: '"Perhaps they are not the stars. But rather openings in the heavens where the love of our lost ones pours through. And shines down upon us to let us know they are happy". We were both touched by the way each square was individualised for their child, just as each of our children is different.' – Gilly and Ruby. Courtesy of The Compassionate Friends (TCF), an organisation of bereaved parents and their families.

Memorial Quilt, Scotland, 2004, originated by Gilly Thomson and Ruby Henderson. Courtesy of The Compassionate Friends (TCF), an organisation of bereaved parents and their families (www.tcf.org.uk/)

Part II

Death and Dying in Poetry, Fiction and the Media

Introduction

Sarah Earle and Carol Komaromy

Death and dying are richly represented in poetry, fiction and the media. Some representations are deeply and profoundly felt personal accounts of impending death or the experience of bereavement. Others seek to provide structure and order to the way in which death and dying can be understood. These, and other forms of representation, can be seen in the selection of pieces presented here.

Part II begins with an extract from the book *The Five People You Meet in Heaven* by Mitch Albom. While the subject of death and dying in literature is approached from many different standpoints, this book explores the concept of 'heaven' and in the dedication to this book Albom notes, 'Everyone has an idea of heaven . . . The version represented here is only a guess, a wish . . .'. Children's fiction, too, often explores the theme of death and dying. The next contribution is an edited extract from the book *Vicky Angel* by Jacqueline Wilson, which tells the story of a girl's best friend who dies suddenly in a car accident. It offers a possibility of hope to those who experience grief for the first time and in this way highlights the role of literature as a powerful form of support.

In the selection of contributions that follow these, attention turns to the themes of mortality and loss. In contrast to the acceptance of the inevitability of death that resonates in romantic poetry, the poem by Dylan Thomas *Do not go gentle into that good night* adopts a much-quoted resistance to the event of death. Also see *Ode to a Nightingale* by John Keats and Wystan Hugh Auden's *Funeral Blues*, which explores loss and bereavement (the latter now well-known after its recital in the film *Four Weddings and a Funeral*). In

Diary Notes, a newly commissioned poem by Jenny Hockey in which her dilemma about going on holiday at the time of her father's illness is powerfully expressed.

War has inspired and continues to inspire writing on the subject of death, dying and bereavement. Contributions here include anti-war poetry by Wilfred Owen and Siegfried Sassoon, as well as a newly commissioned poem again by Jenny Hockey, *Placing the Dead.* Also included is an edited extract from the famous satirical novel *Catch 22* by Joseph Heller, which is set in the later stages of World War II. In contrast to the anti-war poems by the First World War poets represented above, *Catch 22* uses humour and ridicule to show the futility of war.

The next two contributions explore the relationship between illness, sexuality and death in later life. In a two-part poem, a piece of prosetry in *For Phyllis* and *Blind Date*, Yasmin Gutnaratnam is deliberately provocative. Extending the theme of sexuality by exploring the representation of death in the media, Jacque Lynn Foltyn asks: 'Is death the new sex?' Here the author explores the role of the corpse as a commodity in mass entertainment.

The final focus of Part II is on the obituary – a posthumous account of the life of someone who has recently died. Here, the obituary for Dame Cicely Saunders – the founder of the modern hospice movement – who died on 14 July 2005 has been included.

19

The Five People You Meet in Heaven

Mitch Albom

Everyone has an idea of heaven, as do most religions, and they should all be respected. The version represented here is only a guess, a wish.

This is a story about a man named Eddie and it begins at the end, with Eddie dying in the sun. It might seem strange to start a story with an ending. But all endings are also beginnings. We just don't know it at the time.

[…]

Here are the sounds of Eddie's last minutes on earth. Waves crashing. The distant thump of rock music. The whirring engine of a small biplane, dragging an ad from its tail. And this.

"OH MY GOD! LOOK!"

Eddie felt his eyes dart beneath his lids. Over the years, he had come to know every noise at Ruby Pier and could sleep through them all like a lullaby.

This voice was not in the lullaby.

"OH MY GOD! LOOK!"

Eddie bolted upright. A woman with fat, dimpled arms was holding a shopping bag and pointing and screaming. A small crowd gathered around her, their eyes to the skies.

Eddie saw it immediately. Atop Freddy's Free Fall, the new "tower drop" attraction, one of the carts was tilted at an angle, as if trying to dump its cargo. Four passengers, two men, two women, held only by a safety bar, were grabbing frantically at anything they could.

"OH MY GOD!" the fat woman yelled. "THOSE PEOPLE! THEY'RE GONNA FALL!"

[…]

"Don't release the CART!" Eddie yelled. He waved his arms. "HEY! HEEEEY! IT'S THE CABLE! DON'T RELEASE THE CART! IT'LL SNAP!"

The crowd drowned him out. It cheered wildly as Willie and Dominguez unloaded the final rider. All four were safe. They hugged atop the platform.

[…]

Eddie turned to the crowd. "GET BACK!"

Something in Eddie's voice must have caught the people's attention; they stopped cheering and began to scatter. An opening cleared around the bottom of Freddy's Free Fall.

And Eddie saw the last face of his life.

She was sprawled upon the ride's metal base, as if someone had knocked her into it, her nose running, tears filling her eyes, […] Amy? Annie?

Excerpts from *The Five People You Meet in Heaven*, by Mitch Albom, Time Warner, 2004.

"Ma … Mom … Mom …" she heaved, almost rhythmically, her body frozen in the paralysis of crying children.

"Ma … Mom … Ma … Mom … "

Eddie's eyes shot from her to the carts. Did he have time? Her to the carts–

Whump. Too late. The carts were dropping – *Jesus, he released the brake!* – and for Eddie, everything slipped into watery motion. He dropped his cane and pushed off his bad leg and felt a shot of pain that almost knocked him down. A big step. Another step. Inside the shaft of Freddy's Free Fall, the cable snapped its final thread and ripped across the hydraulic line. Cart No. 2 was in a dead drop now, nothing to stop it, a boulder off a cliff.

In those final moments, Eddie seemed to hear the whole world: Distant screaming, waves, music, rush of wind, a low, loud, ugly sound that he realized was his own voice blasting through his chest. The little girl raised her arms. Eddie lunged. His bad leg buckled. He half flew, half stumbled toward her, landing on the metal platform, which ripped through his shirt and split open his skin. […] He felt two hands in his own, two small hands.

A stunning impact.

A blinding flash of light.

And then, nothing.

[*The following extract is taken from the end of the story, when Eddie encounters a little girl whose life he accidentally took, unknowingly, during World War II. He encounters her only again in heaven at the end of the journey.*]

Eddie slumped in the rushing water. The stones of his stories were all around him now, beneath the surface, one touching another. He could feel his form melting, dissolving, and he sensed that he did not have long, that whatever came after the five people you meet in heaven, it was upon him now.

"Tala?" he whispered.

She looked up.

"The little girl at the pier? Do you know about her?"

Tala stared at her fingertips. She nodded yes.

"Did I save her? Did I pull her out of the way?"

Tala shook her head. "No pull."

Eddie shivered. His head dropped. So there it was. The end of his story.

"Push," Tala said.

He looked up. "Push!"

"Push her legs. No pull. You push. Big thing fall. You keep her safe."

Eddie shut his eyes in denial. "But I felt her hands," he said. "It's the only thing I remember. I *couldn't* have pushed her. I felt her *hands*."

Tala smiled and scooped up river water, then placed her small wet fingers in Eddie's adult grip. He knew right away they had been there before.

"Not *her* hands," she said. "Those were *my* hands. I bring you to heaven. Keep you safe."

With that, the river rose quickly, engulfing Eddie's waist and chest and shoulders. Before he could take another breath, the noise of the children disappeared above him, and he was submerged in a strong but silent current. His grip was still entwined with Tala's, but he felt his body being washed from his soul, meat from the bone, and with it went all the pain and weariness he ever held inside him, every scar, every wound, every bad memory.

He was nothing now, a leaf in the water, and she pulled him gently, through shadow and light, through shades of blue and ivory and lemon and black, and he realized all these colors, all along, were the emotions of his life. She drew him up through the breaking waves of a great gray ocean and he emerged in brilliant light above an almost unimaginable scene:

There was a pier filled with thousands of people, men and women, fathers and mothers and children – so many children – children from the past and the present, children who had not yet been born, side by side, hand in hand, in caps, in short pants, filling the boardwalk and the rides and the wooden platforms, sitting on each other's shoulders, sitting in each other's laps. They were there, or would be there, because of the simple, mundane things Eddie had done in his life, the accidents he had prevented, the rides he had kept safe, the unnoticed turns he had affected every day. And while their lips did not move, Eddie heard their voices, more voices than he could have imagined, and a peace came upon him that he had never known before. He was free of Tala's grasp now, and he floated up above the sand and above the boardwalk, above the tent tops and spires of the midway, toward the peak of the big, white Ferris wheel, where a cart, gently swaying, held a woman in a yellow dress – his wife, Marguerite, waiting with her arms extended. He reached for her and he saw her smile and the voices melded into a single word from God:

Home.

20
Vicky Angel
Jacqueline Wilson

I can't take it in. It's not happening. It's some crazy dream. All I need do is blink and I'll wake up in bed and I'll tell Vicky.

Vicky Vicky Vicky Vicky Vicky

I'm running to her.

She's lying in front of the car, face down. Her long red hair is hiding her. I kneel beside her and touch her hand.

[...]

Vicky, I brush her hair back with my shaky hand. Her face in turned sideways. It looks just the same – not a mark. Her mouth could almost be smiling. She has to be all right. This is one of Vicky's little games. She'll sit up in a second and scream with laughter.

[...]

The ambulance woman is checking Vicky's breathing, opening her eyes, shining a torch.

I peer in Vicky's eyes too. The gleam isn't there. I don't think she can see me.

'It's me, Vicky. Jade. Vicky, please be all right. You've got to be OK. Promise me you'll get better. I'll look after you. I'll stay at the hospital. Vicky, I'll do the fun running if you still want, but we don't have to join the Drama Club. I'm probably kidding myself, I'd be useless as an actress. I don't care. The only thing I care about is you. I just want you to be all right, Vicky. You won't die, will you? You can't leave me on my own. I love you, Vic. I love you so much.'

[...]

'You've got a long life, Vicky. Remember the two husbands and all the children?' I remind her, squeezing her hand. She doesn't squeeze back. She lies there, her face pale, her eyes shut, her mouth slightly open as if she's about to say something – but she stays silent.

I'm the one who talks all the way to the hospital, holding her hand tight, but I have to let go when we arrive outside Casualty. I run along beside her until she's suddenly wheeled right away from me by an urgent medical team.

I'm left, lost.

A nurse talks to me. She's asking me my name but I'm in such a muddle I give her Vicky's name instead, Vicky's address, as if Vicky has taken me over completely. I only realize what I've done when she gives me a cup of tea and says 'Here, drink this, Vicky.'

My teeth clink on the china.

'I'm not Vicky,' I say, and I start to cry. [...]

[...]

[...] Vicky's mum and dad suddenly run into Casualty. Mrs Waters has come straight from her aerobics class. She's still in her shocking pink leotard with someone else's too-big tracksuit trousers pulled on top for decency. Mr Waters is still wearing his yellow hard hat from the building site. They gaze round desperately and then see me.

'Jade! Oh God, where's Vicky? We got the message. Is she badly hurt? What *happened*?'

'She got knocked over by a car. I ... she stepped out – she just went straight into it,' I gabble. I hear the squeal of brakes and that one high-pitched scream.

The scream won't stop in my head. It's so loud maybe everyone else can hear it too.

[...]

Vicky's mum is staring at me.

'Did you get knocked down too, Jade?'

I shake my head.

'It was just Vicky. Like I said, she dashed out—'

'Couldn't you have stopped her?'

She doesn't wait for an answer. She runs after Mr Waters. I stand still. I don't know I'm crying until the nurse comes back and presses a wad of paper hankies into my palm.

'There, now, don't worry. She didn't mean it.' [...]

'Mr and Mrs Waters – I wonder, would you come into my office, please?'

I open my eyes. It's another nurse, and a young doctor, a tired-looking guy with lank greasy hair. Poor Vicky, she'll have hoped for a George Clooney look-alike.

I don't know why they're going into the office. To discuss Vicky's treatment? Maybe they want to try an operation? I watch them go and then close my eyes and try bargaining. The rituals get crazier. I have to count to 100 and then stand up, turn round, sit down, another 100, more standing, turning, sitting, *another* 100 ... I must look mad but who cares? Anyway, I can pretend I'm just stretching my legs. If I can make it to a 1000 uninterrupted then Vicky might just be all right. [...]

'Jade.' It's the nurse again.

'No,' I say, shaking my head. Eighty-one, eighty-two, nearly there, eighty-three ...

'Jade, our Vicky, she didn't make it,' Mr Waters sobs.

I know what he means. Of course I do. But I can't let it mean that.

'She didn't make what?' I say.

Mrs Waters gives a little groan. He puts his arm round her.

'I'm afraid Vicky died,' the nurse says quietly.

I stand there, shaking my head, my fists clenched. If I utterly refuse to believe it then maybe it won't have happened.

[...]

'Vicky can't be dead,' I whisper.

'I know it must be so hard to take in. But it's true.'

'She's just in a coma. You look dead in a coma.'

'Darling, we've done all the tests. Vicky's dead.'

'Why can't you put her on a life support machine? Or do that stuff with paddles and shock her back to life?'

'The medical team worked desperately hard. They did everything. Everyone wanted Vicky to live. But she had really bad internal injuries – and then she had a heart attack – no-one could save her. We were all very, very sad.'

'I want to see her.'

'I'm afraid you can't, pet. You're not a relative.'

'I'm like her sister.'

'I know, I know.'

'You don't know. No-one knows. No-one but Vicky.'

[…]

There's a clump of people all around the school gates. What are they looking at? There by the side of the road, right where Vicky lay, is a bunch of red roses. It's as if any split blood has been magically morphed into sweet-smelling flowers.

I stand still, swaying, staring at the bouquet. Someone has written a message: FOR VICKY. I WILL ALWAYS REMEMBER YOU. Vicky's only been dead an hour and yet she's already a memory.

'Wow! I've always wanted a big bunch of red roses,' says Vicky.

I whirl round. There she is, right behind me, her long hair blowing in the breeze. My Vicky. Really.

She grins at my expression.

'You look as if you've seen a ghost!' she says, and then cracks up laughing.

'I don't believe it!'

'What do you think it's like for *me*?' says Vicky. 'It's bad enough when you see a ghost. It's much odder *being* one.'

[…]

21
Do Not Go Gentle Into That Good Night
Dylan Thomas

Do not go gentle into that good night,
Old age should burn and rave at close of day;
Rage, rage against the dying of the light.

Though wise men at their end know dark is right,
Because their words had forked no lightning they
Do not go gentle into that good night.

Good men, the last wave by, crying how bright
Their frail deeds might have danced in a green bay,
Rage, rage against the dying of the light.

Wild men who caught and sang the sun in flight,
And learn, too late, they grieved it on it's way,
Do not go gentle into that good night.

Grave men, near death, who see with blinding sight
Blind eyes could blaze like meteors and be gay,
Rage, rage against the dying of the light.

And you, my father, there on the sad height,
Curse, bless, me now with your fierce tears, I pray.
Do not go gentle into that good nigh.
Rage, rage against the dying of the light.

22
Ode to a Nightingale

John Keats

My heart aches, and a drowsy numbness pains
  My sense, as though of hemlock I had drunk,
Or emptied some dull opiate to the drains
  One minute past, and Lethe-wards had sunk:
'Tis not through envy of thy happy lot,
  But being too happy in thine happiness,—
      That thou, light-wingèd Dryad of the trees,
          In some melodious plot
  Of beechen green, and shadows numberless,
      Singest of summer in full-throated ease.

O, for a draught of vintage! that hath been
  Cool'd a long age in the deep-delved earth,
Tasting of Flora and the country green,
  Dance, and Provençal song, and sunburnt mirth!
O for a beaker full of the warm South,
  Full of the true, the blushful Hippocrene,
      With beaded bubbles winking at the brim,
          And purple-stainèd mouth;
  That I might drink, and leave the world unseen,
      And with thee fade away into the forest dim:

Fade far away, dissolve, and quite forget
  What thou among the leaves hast never known,
The weariness, the fever, and the fret
  Here, where men sit and hear each other groan;
Where palsy shakes a few, sad, last gray hairs,
  Where youth grows pale, and spectre-thin, and dies;
      Where but to think is to be full of sorrow
          And leaden-eyed despairs,
  Where Beauty cannot keep her lustrous eyes,
      Or new Love pine at them beyond to-morrow.

Away! away! for I will fly to thee,
  Not charioted by Bacchus and his pards,
But on the viewless wings of Poesy,
  Though the dull brain perplexes and retards:

'Ode to a nightingale' [final three verses] by John Keats, p.190, Dent & Sons Ltd.

Already with thee! tender is the night,
  And haply the Queen-Moon is on her throne,
    Cluster'd around by all her starry Fays;
      But here there is no light,
  Save what from heaven is with the breezes blown
    Through verdurous glooms and winding mossy ways.

I cannot see what flowers are at my feet,
  Nor what soft incense hangs upon the boughs,
But, in embalmed darkness, guess each sweet
  Wherewith the seasonable month endows
The grass, the thicket, and the fruit-tree wild;
  White hawthorn, and the pastoral eglantine;
    Fast fading violets cover'd up in leaves;
      And mid-May's eldest child,
  The coming musk-rose, full of dewy wine,
    The murmurous haunt of flies on summer eves.

Darkling I listen; and, for many a time
  I have been half in love with easeful Death,
Call'd him soft names in many a mused rhyme,
  To take into the air my quiet breath;
Now more than ever seems it rich to die,
  To cease upon the midnight with no pain,
    While thou art pouring forth thy soul abroad
      In such an ecstasy!
  Still wouldst thou sing, and I have ears in vain—
    To thy high requiem become a sod.

Thou wast not born for death, immortal Bird!
  No hungry generations tread thee down;
The voice I hear this passing night was heard
  In ancient days by emperor and clown:
Perhaps the self-same song that found a path
  Through the sad heart of Ruth, when, sick for home,
    She stood in tears amid the alien corn;
      The same that oft-times hath
  Charm'd magic casements, opening on the foam
    Of perilous seas, in faery lands forlorn.

Forlorn! the very word is like a bell
  To toll me back from thee to my sole self!
Adieu! the fancy cannot cheat so well
  As she is fam'd to do, deceiving elf.
Adieu! adieu! thy plaintive anthem fades
  Past the near meadows, over the still stream,
    Up the hill-side; and now 'tis buried deep
      In the next valley-glades:
  Was it a vision, or a waking dream?
    Fled is that music:—Do I wake or sleep?

23
Funeral Blues

Wystan Hugh Auden

Stop all the clocks, cut off the telephone,
Prevent the dog from barking with a juicy bone,
Silence the pianos and with muffled drum
Bring out the coffin, let the mourners come.

Let aeroplanes circle moaning overhead
Scribbling on the sky the message He is Dead,
Put crêpe bows round the white necks of the public doves,
Let the traffic policemen wear black cotton gloves.

He was my North, my South, my East and West,
My working week and my Sunday rest,
My noon, my midnight, my talk, my song;
I thought that love would last for ever: I was wrong.

The stars are not wanted now: put out every one;
Pack up the moon and dismantle the sun;
Pour away the ocean and sweep up the wood.
For nothing now can ever come to any good.

24
Dairy Notes

Jenny Hockey

Feel we owe him another visit before the holiday.

Flattened throughout July. At times depressed. Hard to form
a smile. Overworked. Desperate to go away. What about
justice? Is there no end to demands too costly to meet? Is
there no-one to say when a break is due? Must take the holiday.

Late July and someone rings. Worried. About him.
His jacket is hanging off. He is confused. His neighbour
confirms it. The doctor suspects malignancy. He has broken
his appointment on June 3rd. Along with two more.

Cigarettes and gin and tonic from the bar. Quickly. Why am I
sailing so far away from someone who is likely to leave me
altogether? Watch the shoreline recede, the deepening of waters.
This holiday is madness. We do not carry a mobile phone.

Approach the Burgundy village and contact. Is he already
dead? The wrong phone number was left. But he is alive
and angry. Somebody passed on information. Someone said he was
ill. And phoned his doctor behind his back. Leave for Rully.

Fifteen weeks later and he is dressed in something blue
and frilly. Which connects directly to the coffin sides. A coverlet
posing as a garment. His hands are visible again. Now utterly
familiar. The red marks on their backs, left behind by the tubes.

Had him briefly. And then he slipped through my fingers.

25

Anthem for Doomed Youth

Wilfred Owen

What passing-bells for these who die as cattle?
  Only the monstrous anger of the guns.
  Only the stuttering rifles' rapid rattle
Can patter out their hasty orisons.
No mockeries for them from prayers or bells,
  Nor any voice of mourning save the choirs,—
The shrill, demented choirs of wailing shells;
  And bugles calling for them from sad shires.

What candles may be held to speed them all?
  Not in the hands of boys, but in their eyes
Shall shine the holy glimmers of good-byes.
  The pallor of girls' brows shall be their pall;
Their flowers the tenderness of silent minds,
And each slow dusk a drawing-down of blinds.

Wilfred Owen, 'Anthem for doomed youth', from John Stallworthy, ed., *Wilfred Owen: The War Poems* (London: Chatto & Windus, 1994). Reprinted with permission.

26
Aftermath
Siegfried Sassoon

Have you forgotten yet? ...
For the world's events have rumbled on since those gagged days,
Like traffic checked while at the crossing of city-ways:
And the haunted gap in your mind has filled with thoughts that flow
Like clouds in the lit heaven of life; and you're a man reprieved to go,
Taking your peaceful share of Time, with joy to spare.
But the past is just the same—and War's a bloody game ...
Have you forgotten yet? ...
Look down, and swear by the slain of the War that you'll never forget.

Do you remember the dark months you held the sector at Mametz—
The nights you watched and wired and dug and piled sandbags on parapets?
Do you remember the rats; and the stench
Of corpses rotting in front of the front-line trench—
And dawn coming, dirty-white, and chill with a hopeless rain?
Do you ever stop and ask, 'Is it all going to happen again?'

Do you remember that hour of din before the attack—
And the anger, the blind compassion that seized and shook you then
As you peered at the doomed and haggard faces of your men?
Do you remember the stretcher-cases lurching back
With dying eyes and lolling heads—those ashen-grey
Masks of the lads who once were keen and kind and gay?

Have you forgotten yet? ...
Look up, and swear by the green of the spring that you'll never forget.

March 1919.

27
Placing the Dead

Jenny Hockey

Photographs that are now all mine,
the beginnings of a classificatory exercise:
Two Edwardian grandmothers, ankle-sock schooldays,
weddings and wars, picnics, babies and beaches,
cardboard studio architecture of immense splendour,
dim glaciers, battalions, the Holy Land,
all my dead, my dead and never once encountered,
family who lost their lives in foreign fields, their battles
with cancer, their freedom from pain. Lost touch.

Up to a high shelf which rests above my office door,
to a legacy of jewellery boxes and attaché cases
I take my ignorance of where they lived and died,
whether they were radiant in their later years and
what sound their voices had. I ask what they did
of a Sunday and what their neighbours thought of it,
how they felt when their sons and husbands were
conscripted. When the War Office Telegram was delivered
what happened to their grief, what became of their love?
Coming down I scrub their dust out of my finger tips
and dream bloody vengeance for their ancient killing.

28
Catch 22
Joseph Heller

[…] "There are some relatives here to see you. Oh, don't worry," he added with a laugh. "Not your relatives. It's the mother, father and brother of that chap who died. They've traveled all the way from New York to see a dying soldier, and you're the handiest one we've got."

"What are you talking about?" Yossarian asked suspiciously. "I'm not dying."

"Of course you're dying. We're all dying. Where the devil else do you think you're heading?"

"They didn't come to see me," Yossarian objected. "They came to see their son."

"They'll have to take what they can get. As far as we're concerned, one dying boy is just as good as any other, or just as bad. To a scientist, all dying boys are equal. I have a proposition for you. You let them come in and look you over for a few minutes and I won't tell anyone you've been lying about your liver symptoms."

Yossarian drew back from him farther. "You know about that?"

"Of course I do. Give us some credit." The doctor chuckled amiably and lit another cigarette. "How do you expect anyone to believe you have a liver condition if you keep squeezing the nurses tits every time you get a chance? You're going to have to give up sex if you want to convince people you've got an ailing liver."

"That's a hell of a price to pay just to keep alive. Why didn't you turn me in if you knew I was faking?"

"Why the devil should I?" asked the doctor with a flicker of surprise. "We're all in this business of illusion together. I'm always willing to lend a helping hand to a fellow conspirator along the road to survival if he's willing to do the same for me. These people have come a long way, and I'd rather not disappoint them. I'm sentimental about old people."

"But they came to see their son."

"They came too late. Maybe they won't even notice the difference."

"Suppose they start crying."

"They probably will start crying. That's one of the reasons they came. I'll listen outside the door and break it up if it starts getting tacky."

"It all sounds a bit crazy," Yossarian reflected. "What do they want to watch their son die for, anyway?"

"I've never been able to figure that one out," the doctor admitted, "but they always do. Well, what do you say? All you've got to do is lie there a few minutes and die a little. Is that asking so much?"

"All right," Yossarian gave in. "If it's just for a few minutes and you promise to wait right outside." He warmed to his role. "Say, why don't you wrap a bandage around me for effect?"

"That sounds like a splendid idea," applauded the doctor.

They wrapped a batch of bandages around Yossarian. A team of medical orderlies installed tan shades on each of the two windows and lowered them to douse the room in depressing shadows.

Yossarian suggested flowers, and the doctor sent an orderly out to find two small bunches of fading ones with a strong and sickening smell. When everything was in place, they made Yossarian get back into bed and lie down. Then they admitted the visitors.

The visitors entered uncertainly as though they felt they were intruding, tiptoeing in with stares of meek apology, first the grieving mother and father, then the brother, a glowering heavy-set sailor with a deep chest. The man and woman stepped into the room stiffly side by side as though right out of a familiar, though esoteric, anniversary daguerreotype on a wall. They were both short, sere and proud. They seemed made of iron and old, dark clothing. The woman had a long, brooding oval face of burnt umber, with coarse graying black hair parted severely in the middle and combed back austerely behind her neck without curl, wave or ornamentation. Her mouth was sullen and sad, her lined lips compressed. The father stood very rigid and quaint in a double-breasted suit with padded shoulders that were much too tight for him. He was broad and muscular on a small scale and had a magnificently curled silver mustache on his crinkled face. His eyes were creased and rheumy, and he appeared tragically ill at ease as he stood awkwardly with the brim of his black felt fedora held in his two brawny laborer's hands out in front of his wide lapels. Poverty and hard work had inflicted iniquitous damage on both. The brother was looking for a fight. His round white cap was cocked at an insolent tilt, his hands were clenched, and he glared at everything in the room with a scowl of injured truculence.

The three creaked forward timidly, holding themselves close to each other in a stealthy, funereal group and inching forward almost in step, until they arrived at the side of the bed and stood staring down at Yossarian. There was a gruesome and excruciating silence that threatened to endure forever. Finally Yossarian was unable to bear it any longer and cleared his throat. The old man spoke at last.

"He looks terrible," he said.

"He's sick, Pa."

"Giuseppe," said the mother, who had seated herself in a chair with her veinous fingers clasped in her lap.

"My name is Yossarian," Yossarian said.

"His name is Yossarian, Ma. Yossarian, don't you recognize me? I'm your brother John. Don't you know who I am?"

"Sure I do. You're my brother John."

"He does recognize me! Pa, he knows who I am. Yossarian, here's Papa. Say hello to Papa."

"Hello, Papa," said Yossarian.

"Hello, Giuseppe."

"His name is Yossarian, Pa."

"I can't get over how terrible he looks," the father said.

"He's very sick, Pa. The doctor says he's going to die."

"I didn't know whether to believe the doctor or not," the father said. "You know how crooked those guys are."

"Giuseppe," the mother said again, in a soft, broken chord of muted anguish.

"His name is Yossarian, Ma. She don't remember things too good any more. How're they treating you in here, kid? They treating you pretty good?"

"Pretty good," Yossarian told him.

"That's good. Just don't let anybody in here push you around. You're just as good as anybody else in here even though you are Italian. You've got rights, too."

Yossarian winced and closed his eyes so that he would not have to look at his brother John. He began to feel sick.

"*Now* see how terrible he looks," the father observed.

"Giuseppe," the mother said.

"Ma, his name is Yossarian," the brother interrupted her impatiently. "Can't you remember?"

"It's all right," Yossarian interrupted him. "She can call me Giuseppe if she wants to."

"Giuseppe," she said to him.

"Don't worry, Yossarian," the brother said. "Everything is going to be all right."

"Don't worry, Ma," Yossarian said. "Everything is going to be all right."

"Did you have a priest?" the brother wanted to know.

"Yes," Yossarian lied, wincing again.

"That's good," the brother decided. "Just as long as you're getting everything you've got coming to you. We came all the way from New York. We were afraid we wouldn't get here in time."

"In time for what?"

"In time to see you before you died."

"What difference would it make?"

"We didn't want you to die by yourself."

"What difference would it make?"

"He must be getting delirious," the brother said. "He keeps saying the same thing over and over again."

"That's really very funny," the old man replied. "All the time I thought his name was Giuseppe, and now I find out his name is Yossarian. That's really very funny."

"Ma, make him feel good," the brother urged. "Say something to cheer him up."

"Giuseppe."

"It's not Giuseppe, Ma. It's Yossarian."

"What difference does it make?" the mother answered in the same mourning tone, without looking up. "He's dying."

Her tumid eyes filled with tears and she began to cry, rocking back and forth slowly in her chair with her hands lying in her lap like fallen moths. Yossarian was afraid she would start wailing. The father and brother began crying also. Yossarian remembered suddenly why they were all crying, and he began crying too. A doctor Yossarian had never seen before stepped inside the room and told the visitors courteously that they had to go. The father drew himself up formally to say goodbye.

"Giuseppe," he began.

"Yossarian," corrected the son.

"Yossarian," said the father.

"Giuseppe," corrected Yossarian.

"Soon you're going to die."

Yossarian began to cry again. The doctor threw him a dirty look from the rear of the room, and Yossarian made himself stop.

The father continued solemnly with his head lowered. "When you talk to the man upstairs," he said, "I want you to tell Him something for me. Tell Him it ain't right for people to die when they're young. I mean it. Tell Him if they got to die at all, they got to die when they're old. I want you to tell Him that. I don't think He knows it ain't right, because He's supposed to be good and it's been going on for a long, long time. Okay?"

"And don't let anybody up there push you around," the brother advised. "You'll be just as good as anybody else in heaven, even though you are Italian."

"Dress warm," said the mother, who seemed to know.

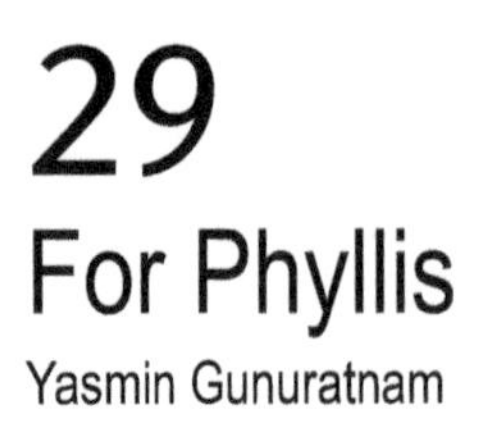

29
For Phyllis

Yasmin Gunuratnam

Phyllis Dourado. Femme-fatale.

She called herself a girl.

I can see her now, standing at the top of her stairs in her house-coat and pearls, hair still suggestive of the curlers that had only recently been removed. Her face thick with make-up. Mask-like. Powder, a shade too chalky for her brown skin. Green eye-shadow. Pink lipstick. Come to think of it, I am not sure that I ever saw Phyllis without her make-up.

We're Roman Catholic, she told me with pride, the first time that we met. I pray quite often, and I always have faith, even if something is, um, beyond my reach. I still have that small bit of faith floating around. But I don't seem to be able to finish my prayers these days. Too many questions go around in my mind. Why has this happened to me? What have I done to deserve this? I don't know, my mind is so troubled.

The next time I saw Phyllis, in her neat, semi-detached house, she stood up in mid-sentence, moved slowly across the room, sat down next to me and leaned forward. Our heads were almost touching. The troubles that I told you about before, she whispered, it's my boyfriend. He's married.

Not only married. The husband of her best friend. A thirty-year love affair.

Thirty years of nervous distraction. Edgy expectation every time the telephone rang, or mail plunged helplessly onto the door-mat, or a car pulled up outside the house. Always in a state of readiness, Phyllis had taken to plumping up the cushions of denial that lay scattered strategically throughout her home.

And do you know what? Phyllis said out loud, hugging a cushion to her breast, I can't come to grips with not ever being with this guy, like I can't come to grips with this cancer.

Hope and hopelessness. Sitting right next to each other. Almost touching.

Is it possible to be terminally sexy? Still hopeful of love on your death-bed?

Still so much a girl?

30
Blind Date

Yasmin Gunuratnam

Sixty-five and so alive
with cancer.
Grasped in the passionate arms of a metastatic spread
that outdoes the erotic devotion of my most ardent
and agile of lovers.
Sometimes just the merest suggestion of a
touch.
Takes my breath away.
Makes my back arch.
Leaves me wondering if it is all a dream.
Sometimes a desperate, urgent embrace.
Off the Richter-scale of the tactile
Demanding immediate recognition. Eternal fidelity.

The thrill, I am told, lies in the chase.
I am tired of the games.
Catch me.

Furtive encounters beneath the skin.
Right underneath the doctor's nose.
I call that kinky.

Like mango pulp eaten off my stomach.
In the afternoon.

Like there is no tomorrow.
No space here for these messy, subcutaneous entanglements
Death and desire.
Instead, on a plate, I am offered 'Think Positive'.
'Take Each Day As it Comes'.

Tiresome conspiracies,
prepare a bed made ready for self-betrayal and blame.
Keeping it manageable. Tidy. Clean.

I am here to lower the tone.
I like it dirty.
Eat me.
So walk with me into the back-row of life.
Kiss me slowly into oblivion.
I am not interested in the show.
I am here to be caressed. Cradled. Enfolded.
                    The ultimate X-rated embrace.

No more fleshy denial.
No more refusals.
I want to open up. Feel the stickiness of this intimacy
                                        that is not invasion,

to twist and writhe my way through your rhizomatic routes
To just this side of rapture, that is me.
All me.

I am here.
Take me.

So after the morphine, the smile from a face
                            forever held at half tilt,

Pass me my powder.
My rouge. My lipstick.

I can't go out looking
like this.

31
Dead Sexy: Why Death is the New Sex

Jacque Lynn Foltyn

Three years ago, while visiting a friend in Paris, I turned on the television and noticed something surprising. Human remains had moved center stage in France as well as in the US and the UK. As I clicked the remote among forensic detective programs and documentaries about Peruvian and Egyptian mummies, I thought to myself, 'Ah, it's going on here too . . .'

From *CSI: Crime Scene Investigation* to *Actual Autopsy* and *Body Worlds,* Gunther von Hagen's traveling museum exhibit of plastinated human remains, the corpse is the star of the show. *Hannibal* and *The Passion of the Christ* parade the tortured dead as spectacles, while the protagonist of *Kissed* is a female necrophiliac. The reality TV series *Family Plots* showcases cadavers as main characters in a funeral home, while a dead woman narrates *Desperate Housewives.* In 2004, Britain's Science Museum, in conjunction with the UK's Channel 4, proposed the ultimate corpse production: *Dust to Dust,* a series documenting the decomposition of an actual human body.

Natural disasters and war, medical innovations such as cadaver collagen and face transplants, and the international trafficking of body parts have also placed the corpse center stage, I note. Hospital, cemetery, and crematoria scandals in which corpses have been misplaced, discarded as trash, or dismantled and sold as if they were used auto parts have also brought the corpse to the fore.

Feeding pop culture's obsession with forensics, dissection, decay, and DNA, video games are littered with simulations of decomposing bodies. My nephews call them 'cool.' It took me a mere 0.04 seconds to Google 12,400,000 autopsy websites. As I surf the web, I find body bags and fake corpses for sale. 'One can specify the degree of composition desired,' I marvel, while my husband Henry rolls his eyes as I show him an eBay site. Macabre images of dead bodies in morgues are propagating like locusts across media land. The corpse count has gone up on prime time TV, more than double in 2005 of what it was in 2004, according to the Parents Television Council, a US media watchdog body. In our youth and beauty-obsessed culture, dead celebrities are more popular than live ones and any unsolved mystery about the gruesome murder of a pretty young female is a sensation. (So popular are these narratives, the feminist scholar in me is beginning to think they are culturally sanctioned.) Whether fantasy or fact, this is the corpse's cultural moment.

Despite this growing obsession with dead bodies, I note an irony: in western civilization the cadaver remains the body's most polluted form, something to deny, disguise, and hide. Calling them distressing, President Bush forbids the publication of photographs of coffins, returned from Iraq, laden with fallen soldiers. There was international outrage when bootlegged video of Saddam Hussein, swinging from a noose, was available on YouTube shortly after his execution.

Clearly, members of society are of two minds about the corpse, attracted and repulsed by it, viewing it as both sacred and profane.

Looking for answers to this duality, I turn to anthropologist Geoffrey Gorer's essay, *The Pornography of Death* (1955). According to Gorer, popular culture filled a void created by taboos about death in the 20th century, as death exchanged positions with sex as *the* taboo subject. As western societies became more liberated about sex, Gorer reasoned, they rejected death and some of its cultural practices (e.g., lengthy mourning, widow's weeds). Natural death, the dead body, and decomposition became too horrific to contemplate. Taboos against death created a psychologically disturbed mass audience for unnatural, violent deaths as entertainment genre, argued Gorer, a genre he viewed as pornographic because of its brutality, exploitation, and remove from normal emotions like grief. Gorer likened the phenomenon to the pervasiveness of sex pornography and prostitution in the Victorian era, a period when piano legs were thought obscene and covered with curtains.

There is much to value in Gorer's core argument. Far removed from many of our lives, natural death is often sequestered in hospitals and old people's homes, and is geographically isolated, as many family and friends scatter across nations and continents. Death seems off in the distance, a 'failure of a cure,' as the historian Philippe Ariès put it. People may be shocked when someone they know dies, protesting the unfairness of such a fate. My husband, a physician, sees it all of the time in his practice, and does his best to explain to his dying patients and their families that death is normal.

The fact is, many people living in North America and Western Europe have never seen an actual dead person or witnessed a real death. I speak from experience. Before 2005, I viewed death as an abstract problem, not a part of life. That changed when my first husband Matthew died in my arms from cancer, with no family members present save my parents and me, his ex-wife. I remember trying to close Matt's eyes and make his face relax, when a hospice nurse stopped me. 'It's not like you see in the movies,' she explained, gently.

Gorer's argument, while insightful, needs revision for the 21st century. When he wrote his famous essay, there were plenty of pornographic images of dead bodies in popular culture. The good and the bad were strangled, shot, and thrown off buildings; they were gamma-rayed by space aliens, dragged into murky swamps by creatures from the black lagoon, and bitten to death by vampires. *However*, the camera did not linger over these deaths and the images themselves were tame. Bodies fell, the camera moved away, or if the camera focused on the dying or dead body at all, it was whole and appeared to be sleeping, not contorted in death agonies. My thoughts turn back nostalgically to *Quincy, M.E.,* the 1976–1983 medical examiner program. Exploration of the human cadaver and its decomposition were not aims; the cadaver was given privacy, discreetly covered by a sheet on the gurney, with perhaps a big toe with an ID tag sticking out.

I knew Quincy's corpses were not real. Today's fictive corpses are imbued with verisimilitude, designed to appear real in ways that I have no doubt would have shocked Gorer, were he living today. The new pornography of death is as grief-gutted as the old, but dazzles the audience with grisly corpses, flashy forensic technology and exotic causes of death that are far removed from their experience. There is a sense of unreality as well as reality about these corpse shows in which people die from asphyxiation in tar, from stomachs burst while overeating, from accidental decapitation, from being sucked into a tree shredder, or from being eaten alive by insects. This is death at its most ghastly, exploitative, and that is precisely the point of the 21st-century pornography of death. After finding these programs initially informational and interesting, as the carnage factor went up, I found them repugnant, disrespectful, no matter how much warmth and wit was written into the characterizations of the forensics team. After Matt's death, I could not stomach them anymore.

Recently, a theology professor, attending one of my lectures, told me about *Anatomy*, a film chronicling the misadventures of a group of demented doctors who dissect sexy young lovelies and view corpse parts as artworks. 'Death is the mother of beauty,' I muse to myself, remembering the evocative lines of the poet Wallace Stevens. Yes, death is the new sex and never more so than now, when death has not merely supplanted sex as a cultural taboo, but merged with it. Granted, eroticization of the corpse is nothing new. 'My first nude was the erotic body of the dead Christ,' observed a philosopher friend of mine. Artists have long made dead bodies look sexy (e.g., Greek flower myths, Michelangelo's *Dying Slave*, Millais' *Ophelia*, Pabst's *Lulu*, Minghella's *The English Patient;* edgy fashion photography.) The connection of fertility with cycles of sex, death, and rebirth is probably the most widespread of all ritual associations (Napier 1986), and it makes sense that sex and death would mix in our imaginative minds. Freud understood this when he speculated that death and sexual beauty share a 'hidden identity.'

As taboos about both sex and death have relaxed, a growing conflation of the two once forbidden bodies, the sex body and the dead body, can be seen. If the unmourned, unnatural, violent death, identified by Gorer, is one kind of pornography of death; and the focus on the appalling corpse, I discuss, another; I believe a third kind of death pornography has emerged in contemporary culture that combines the aforementioned two and sexualizes them. Hence, the decomposing, mutilated, young, gorgeous victims of unnatural, violent deaths from kinky sexual practices or from the hands of sexual sadists. (On one memorable episode of *Medium*, an attractive young woman dies from shock, tied to a chair, after her face is sliced into a grotesque mask.) Designed to highlight the body's sexuality as well as its decomposition, *corpse porn*, as I call it, transforms the dead body in theatrical ways, designed to disturb and titillate. The forensic lab invites our eyes to linger, presenting death as an enticing sight, as corpses of beautiful—or once beautiful—young people lie mute on slabs in morgues (which may have atmospheric lighting and mood music), waiting for investigators to make their bodies 'speak' of secret vices, criminal passions, and, of course, victimization.

While the word 'pornography' is bandied about rather loosely these days, and definitions of what is obscene are culturally and historically relative, I contend that the word remains appropriate when examining the phenomenon I am describing. The corpse is pop culture's latest porn star, the new body voyeuristically explored. Corpse porn and sex porn have more in common than one might expect. Both exploit the nude, young, the whole, and the beautiful, not the clothed, the old, the diseased, and the ugly. Both rely on the close-up, the detailed exploration of every nook and cranny of the body, which is prodded, poked, penetrated, and presented as an outrageous sight. Both luxuriate in body fluids. Viewers watch and listen as CSI teams discuss penile implants, pierced clitorises, missing nipples, S&M lash marks, and obscene tattoos in places where the sun does not shine. Socially appropriate emotion is absent from both kinds of pornography. Love from sex porn. Grief, reflection, and discussion of the preciousness of life from corpse porn, which divorces the dead body from spiritual or other moral lessons such as compassion. Each moves easily into camp, especially in their American versions, with their kitschy plot lines, bantering detectives and coroners, and double-entendres. Moreover, while the corpse porn star just as the sex porn star is most often a female, because of woman's closer association with birth, sex, death, and dirt (de Beauvoir 1974; Douglas 1966), neither today is woman's exclusive iconographic domain.

In a 2006 episode of *Law & Order: Criminal Intent*, an emblematic corpse porn plot is screened. A dead woman is found by surfers, and is revealed to have fallen from a jet wheel, where she had been stuffed post-mortem. Viewers learn that she had been a sex slave, held captive in a soundproof room, chained to a wall and let loose only to participate in boxing matches with a man, who is sexually aroused by beating women to death, who is watched by another man who is sexually aroused by watching the other man beat women to death. Along the way, viewers watch a female detective lift the sheet covering the poor woman's body and note that she has piercings in her labia.

Not so long ago, I was walking with my old friend Charles, 88, an English historian, and described this macabre plot. Aghast, he stopped in his tracks, shook his head, and exclaimed, 'How disgusting that our culture has sunk to this new low of depravity!' If one agrees with Charles that corpse porn marks a new cultural low, or prefers, instead, simply to concede that macabre death and corpses have become common entertainment fare, the question remains: Why?

I have been studying representations of dead bodies since 1993, and have watched, fascinated, as the corpse has risen as an infotainment commodity, a hybrid of information and entertainment. Today's electronic media reflects a redistribution of power relations around the dead body, blurring the boundaries between the living and the dead.

Novelty and the drive for ratings tied to advertising revenues are part of the answer, of course. Our popular culture and entertainment industries, exported globally, place primary focus on killing and the degradation of the corpse. Today's popular forensic science programs rely on voyeuristic inspections of the cadaver to solve crimes and transform the corpse into something new: a problem to be solved. This explains why long running crime series like *Law and Order*, which in the past featured an unimpressive corpse for a second or two at the beginning of the show, have added morgues, coroners, and autopsies to their programs, and increasingly bizarre forms of death.

Realistic representations of dead bodies are a novelty in our entertainment, consumer, and information society, reviving the past 'glory' of the pre-modern corpse, when the church and political leaders displayed it to teach moral and political lessons. Pop culture's current corpse is detached from theological and political lessons, and is used instead to stimulate dark fantasies about death, sex, and violence, but in simulated form, i.e., at a distance. Since sex today sells everything from celebrity to Uncle Ben's Rice, why not use it to sell death? In societies oversaturated with images of sex, sexuality has lost some of its allure. Corpse porn jazzes things up, making both the banality of sex and the banality of death new.

The corpse is being recoded, desacralized, and transacted in numerous other ways by those who view the dead body as a worldly commodity to exploit. Genomics, stem cell research, organ harvesting, cross-species transplants, and cloning have expanded the public need to discuss proper 'uses' of the corpse, spurring action by public policy initiators and outcries by moral leaders and an incensed public determined to protect the dead from the living.

A culture's ideas about death are closely related to its ideas about life. Arguably, this is a secular world which emphasizes consumer goods and services, material wealth, entertainment, information, technology, youth, sex, and beauty, all of which are temporal, worldly. In the past, the dead were said to haunt us; today, the living hover around the dead and refuse to let them rest, finding new ways to turn them into commodities. But as attempts are made to transmogrify the corpse into a manageable entertainment, information, and biomedical commodity, not a fearful object reminding us of our own demises, it is easy to forget that that death will not be tamed; it will come for all of us too, and will not be scheduled into a one-hour television slot.

References

de Beauvoir, S. (1974) *The Second Sex: The Classic Manifesto of the Liberated Woman*. New York: Vintage Books.

Douglas, M. (1966) *Purity and Danger: An Analysis of the Concepts of Purity and Taboo*. London: Routledge.

Gorer, G. (1955) 'The pornography of death', *Encounter*, 5, 49–52.

Napier, D.L. (1986) *Masks, Transformations and Paradox*. Berkeley, CA: University of California Press.

32
Obituary: Dame Cicely Saunders

Visionary founder of the modern hospice movement who set the highest standards in care for the dying
The Times
22 June 1918 – 14 July 2005

DAME CICELY SAUNDERS earned gratitude, admiration and international renown for helping to alleviate the suffering of terminally ill people.

Hundreds of hospices in Britain and more than 95 other countries are modelled on St Christopher's, Sydenham, the hospice which she established in 1967.

St Christopher's, on her initiative, attempted for the first time to provide patient-centred palliative care for the terminally ill, combining emotional, spiritual and social support with expert medical and nursing care. Its practices have since been widely copied and developed. Today St Christopher's cares for about 2,000 patients and their families each year and, in training more than 60,000 health professionals, has influenced standards of care for the dying throughout the world.

Despite coming late in life to her vocation – she trained in turn as a nurse, almoner, medical secretary and doctor, before opening St Christopher's – by the time she died Saunders had gained a place in public esteem almost comparable to that occupied by Florence Nightingale.

She had, in fact, begun her training in 1940 as a Nightingale nurse. A shy, tall, gawky young woman, she had felt the need for some stronger wartime commitment than the completion of an Oxford degree – a task to which she returned when a lifelong back defect made a nursing career impossible, before going on to qualify as a hospital social worker. But for all her dedication, much strengthened by her conversion to evangelical Christianity, Saunders was for long uncertain how best to deploy her passionate concern for the sick and suffering.

She was in many ways an old-fashioned woman, a charismatic *grande dame* with strong values and a great talent for leadership. She was such a remarkable innovator in the treatment of physical and psychological pain that she eventually held fellowships in the Royal College of Physicians (1974), the Royal College of Nursing (1981) and the Royal College of Surgeons (1986).

She was awarded the esteemed Templeton, Onassis and Wallenberg prizes, a score of honorary degrees and medals, was advanced from OBE (1967) to DBE in 1980 and appointed to

---

the Order of Merit in 1989. In 2001 she was awarded the million-dollar Conrad N. Hilton Humanitarian Prize.

None of this was easily achieved. Born Cicely Mary Strode Saunders in Barnet, North London, in 1918, she was the eldest daughter of a prosperous, domineering estate agent, whose unhappy marriage to a dependent wife broke up in 1945, the critical year in which Saunders graduated from Oxford and abruptly exchanged the agnosticism in which she had grown up for an earnest religious search for a mission.

She was unhappy at home, even more unhappy at Roedean, eager for a partnership in life which she could not find among her widening circle of colleagues and friends. Seeking a better-matched relationship than her parents, she found it only in middle age, with the émigré Polish painter Marian Bohusz-Szyszko, a Catholic, whom she married in 1980, after the death of his separated wife in Poland.

Other Poles had earlier played a decisive role in her life. Saunders herself wondered why she felt such a lifelong attraction towards things and persons Polish. She attributed much of it to an intimate but unconsummated love for a dying patient, David Tasma, a refugee from the Warsaw ghetto, whom she met on her first rounds as an almoner at St Thomas's. He was a friendless waiter with no family, and there was no consolation for him except in the love which she discovered to be within her reach. It was then that she saw how the pain of cancer could be tamed by modern drugs and that unavoidable distress could be made tolerable by a form of care that ranked the physical and spiritual needs of the patient together.

Tasma bequeathed her all his worldly goods, £500, which she treasured for years until she found a way to give full effect to his cryptic wish that it should be "a window in your home". His gift is now commemorated in the entrance to St Christopher's.

Her experience as a volunteer in St Luke's, the Bayswater Home for the Dying Poor, persuaded Saunders to challenge the received medical wisdom about dying, death and bereavement. She put herself back to school, studied physics and chemistry and qualified as a doctor when she was 38. She then combined membership of a research group on pain, set up at St Mary's, Paddington, with her continuing ward work – this time at St Joseph's Hackney, where the Sisters of Charity showed her how much might be done for the dying by sustained loving care; and where she, in turn, began to bring into play her more unorthodox ideas about pain relief.

What she then demonstrated, and what is now widely adopted, was that intermittent reactive sedation of surging pain was far less effective than achieving a steady state in which the dying patient could still maintain consciousness and even live with some quality.

At St Joseph's Saunders met the second of the Poles who changed her life. The transfiguration of Antoni Michniewicz showed her what dying might be like when love could be given and received. His death inspired her in her plan to found St Christopher's – named, appropriately, after the patron saint of travellers – as a place to find shelter on the most difficult part of life's journey.

St Christopher's was to cater primarily for cancer patients, because Saunders had seen a gap in NHS provision, highlighted by a 1952 Marie Curie Foundation survey of their needs and a later Gulbenkian report on the care of the chronic sick – a perspective which today carries the principles and practice of palliative care beyond the initial concern with cancer.

It took years of planning and financing to open a purpose-built hospice on the Sydenham site. There Saunders explored all the possibilities for matching quality medical care with support for patients and their families at home, changing existing medical and social attitudes about the care of the dying. Through the struggles for financial and professional backing, in which Saunders proved herself as a medical director, a fundraiser of quiet genius, a relentless administrator and a proponent of the hospice idea on the world stage, it was clear that she was achieving exactly what she set out to do.

The change she accomplished in medical attitudes was most notably recognised when the Royal College of Physicians established palliative medicine as a distinct medical specialism.

When the Cicely Saunders Foundation was launched in 2002, her reputation attracted leading specialists from North America and Australia to its international scientific advisory panel. The foundation aims to promote research into all aspects of palliative medicine and care for the dying, with particular emphasis on collaborations between different professions in healthcare, clinical and non-clinical services, to improve the integration between research and practice.

Many years ago, in response to a question at a symposium about the prospect of death, Saunders declared that she would hope for a sudden demise but would prefer to die – as she has – with a cancer that gave due notice and allowed the time to reflect on life and to put one's practical and spiritual affairs in order.

Her husband, Marian Bohusz-Szysko, died in 1995, aged 92.

Dame Cicely Saunders, OM, DBE, the founder of the modern hospice movement, was born on June 22, 1918. She died on July 14, 2005, aged 87.

Part III

Death, Dying and Bereavement on the World Wide Web

Introduction

Sarah Earle and Carol Komaromy

The increasing accessibility of the World Wide Web has transformed the potential for global communication and information-sharing. It is this and its potential to transform practices and relationships in the field of death, dying and bereavement that is the focus of Part III.

Part III begins with an edited extract of a paper that first appeared in the journal *Generations*. This contribution, written by Pamela Roberts, explores the range of ways in which the Web is used to memorialise those who have died and to attain support when bereaved. The author discusses personal web memorials, the web memorial services provided by the funeral industry, funerals broadcast over webcams, and bereavement support on the Web. The next set of contributions provide some examples of these and other ways in which the World Wide Web can transform experiences of death, dying and bereavement. See, for example, the pieces *Winston's Wish: For Young People, Bereavement UK: The Garden of Tranquillity* and *Andrea Rouen's Farewell* as well as the piece *Cancergiggles*, a blog written by a man dying of colon cancer. The web challenges the axes of space and time which are key to the notion of death and loss.

In the next piece, which has been newly commissioned for this volume, Anna Davidsson Bremborg examines the publication of photographs of dead bodies on the Web. Drawing on two distinct examples – the publication of photographs for the purposes of identification following the 2004 Asian Tsunami, and the use of photographs of dead babies on memorialisation websites – the author explores the way in which the World

Wide Web facilitates communication, but also poses new questions about the ethical justification of such use and challenges the practice of the concealment of dead bodies.

Continuing with a focus on the new challenges posed by the widespread use of the World Wide Web, the final contribution in this part of the book looks at the issue of suicide. The piece by Katja Becker and Martin H. Schmidt explore the use of 'suicide web forums' amongst young people with suicidal ideations. Again, this raises ethical issues that have been unprecedented in other communication technologies.

The majority of organisations providing information, support and other services in the area of death, dying and bereavement now have some kind of presence on the World Wide Web. The ease of access that this provides is increasingly realised as demand for this resource grows. A brief annotated list of these is provided at the end of Part III.

33
Here Today and Cyberspace Tomorrow: Memorials and Bereavement Support on the Web

Pamela Roberts

[...]

Personal web memorials

[...] Web memorials allow the bereaved to honor their dead in their own way and at their own time, to visit the memorial whenever they choose, and to share with others memories and information about the deceased person.

Web memorials vary in many ways and are created by a wide range of people with different levels of skill and expertise. The most labor-intensive form of web memorialization is the web page created and posted by bereaved individuals. Because individual memorials are often posted as freestanding web pages, they are difficult for researchers to access. Consequently, we know very little about the frequency with which they are created or the characteristics of the people who create them. However, anecdotal evidence suggests that many people who already have web pages at the time of bereavement create memorial web pages to honor their dead. In some instances, an existing web page is revised to become a memorial. [...]

With no common cultural rules dictating their content, length, or the accepted symbols to employ, web memorials vary according to their creator's tastes, needs, and computer skills. Some memorials are very simple, similar to grave markers, showing a simple graphic (such as a picture of a bouquet) with the person's name and dates of birth and death. On the other hand, some web memorials are elaborate and include music, moving images (for example, angels fluttering their wings), pictures and videos of the dead, and long tributes to them (sometimes the equivalent of several typewritten pages). One memorial starts with the picture of a preschool boy, his birth and death dates, and links to chapters about him. [...] Like many other web memorials, this one has a guest book, where anyone can record messages or read the notes of others.

Freestanding web memorials can be linked together to form "web rings," collections of web pages where one can travel from one web memorial to another. Memorial web rings are most often created for deceased children. [...]

Constructing an individual memorial web page provides freedom of expression and the opportunity to update the memorial at any time, but the process is inaccessible to those without the required computer skills. More accessible are grouped memorial sites such as "web cemeteries," established sites where one can post a memorial, either free or for a fee.

Most web cemeteries (see Roberts, 1999) provide the opportunity for anyone who can use e-mail to create a web memorial. [...]

Much like individual memorial web pages, memorials in most web cemeteries allow the bereaved to honor their dead with few format or content restrictions. Most web cemeteries have standard information at the top of each memorial (usually the name and dates of birth and death), but the rest is created by the bereaved. Consequently, these memorials vary in size and scope. Some contain only a simple phrase like "Rest in Peace" or another short, more individual sentiment; one reads "Finally hung up the hoe." Others have long tributes (sometimes a few typewritten pages) and include poems, links to other websites, and notes from more than one author. Many are letters written to the dead person, while other written postings describe the personal qualities of the deceased, but few include the lists of accomplishments that are common in traditional obituaries (Roberts and Vidal, 2000; de Vries and Rutherford, in press). A typical web memorial might inform the reader that the deceased cooked an excellent barbecue and always did magic tricks for the grandchildren and omit the fact that she was president of the local bank.

Other types of sites also provide opportunities to memorialize the dead. [...] Some websites allow people to memorialize the dead according to the cause of death. For example, one site (The Body, 2004) provides a place for memorializing deaths due to AIDS.

Because web memorials are so new, little is known about the process of creating them. Studies of memorials in web cemeteries have found that the memorials are most often written for family members, especially parents (Roberts and Vidal, 2000; de Vries and Rutherford, in press). Older adults are frequently memorialized; both of the above studies analyzed memorials for individuals in their late 90s. Most web memorials appear to be heartfelt, positively portraying the deceased and noting the author's grief at the person's death. Memorials in web cemeteries put older people in their rightful place, as members of a multiage community in which loss of relationships and distinct personalities is mourned, regardless of the age of the deceased. In so doing, these memorials provide a welcome contrast to the way the culture typically minimizes the impact of the death of older people (Moss, Moss, and Hansson, 2001).

[...]

Web memorialization provides unique, supplemental postdeath rituals for the bereaved. Web memorials, unlike most postdeath rituals, can be created at one's own pace; in our research on early memorials in three web cemeteries, over 7 percent were created for individuals who had died 20 or more years before the memorial was posted (Roberts and Vidal, 2000). Web memorials also can be created by anyone, including friends and others who were not included in standard mourning rituals. Friends are frequently disenfranchised in death (Doka, 1989); posting a web memorial honors the importance of a friendship, which may be overlooked in traditional postdeath rituals. In descriptive studies of web cemeteries, friends posted approximately 15 percent of the memorials (Roberts and Vidal, 2000; de Vries and Rutherford, in press). Web memorials also allow the bereaved to honor relationship that may be undervalued in the general society. For example, some cemeteries accept memorials for pets.

Individual web pages and many memorials in web cemeteries can be changed and updated. In a display of continuing bonds with the dead, one can care for the memorial much like one tends a grave. In addition, web memorials can be visited at any time and from any location.

Visits to web memorials serve functions similar to those of visiting a place of interment. Most of the bereaved visit a web memorial to show their love for the dead and to feel the person's presence (Roberts et al., 2000, 2003). The opportunity to visit a web memorial may be especially valuable to elders with limited mobility, for whom visiting an interment site is difficult.

Web memorials also allow the bereaved to share memories of the deceased and their relationship. Not only can one share the memorial with people who are physically distant, but also many of our survey respondents report sitting in front of the computer screen with others, visiting the memorial together (Roberts et al., 2000, 2003). Such activities promote a sense of closeness and community among bereaved people (Roberts, in press), which may be especially valuable to more isolated elders.

While the research on web memorialization is limited, all indicators suggest that creating web memorials has a positive impact on the bereaved. In both survey studies (Roberts et al., 2000, 2003), all but a few participants said that creating memorials had helped in their bereavement and that they would create another. Some 19 percent of bereaved parents in the survey spontaneously mentioned that they have helped others create web memorials because their own experiences were so beneficial. [...]

Other postdeath rituals

Not long after the creation of web cemeteries and other grouped memorial websites, many in the funeral industry added web memorials to their list of services. At present, most of the memorials provided by mortuaries are created using the FuneralNet Memorial Obituary Program (FuneralNet, 2004). This program incorporates information given by the bereaved into a format that is reminiscent of a traditional obituary. These memorials typically include a picture of the deceased, a description of their accomplishments, a list of survivors, information on funeral services, and a guest book. Missing are the words of the bereaved themselves. Like other web memorials, these tributes can be viewed at any time, by anyone with web access. [...] While these memorials afford greater geographical and temporal access than standard obituaries, the bereaved are so far removed from the process that it is unlikely that these memorials provide the benefits that personal web memorials offer. There is no research on mortuary-created web memorials, but anecdotal reports are not encouraging.

Many mortuaries are branching out into other web-based services. Increasingly popular are funeral services broadcast over a webcam. Such transmissions allow bereaved individuals who cannot travel to the ceremony to attend "virtually." This provision could be of benefit to seniors with mobility problems, allowing them to experience some postdeath rituals in real time.

The Forever Network (2004), a company associated with, but whose clients are not limited to those interred at Hollywood Forever Cemetery, is a pioneer in another increasingly popular service, creating digital movie tributes to the dead. All of those interred in Hollywood Forever are provided a digital tribute, which includes pictures of the dead that are displayed one by one as music plays in the background. Typically the tribute is played at the funeral and then is posted on the web. In addition, the Forever Network creates Life Stories, which include videotaped interviews with relatives, friends, and even the deceased if they made previous arrangements. Life stories are posted on the Network's website with the promise that storage will be updated as new formats become available. Tributes and Life Stories are not only posted on the web, but also can be accessed at several kiosks on the grounds of Hollywood Forever.

[...]

While most of the above services focus on memorialing the dead, others provide peace of mind for the living as they contemplate their own death. For example, My Last Wish (2004) bills itself as an electronic safety deposit box, where the living can store wishes, letters, pictures, and video and sound files that will be delivered to others at the time of one's death.

Thus, there are many types of web services available to help the bereaved memorialize the dead, have greater access to traditional post-death rituals, and to transmit wishes beyond the grave. Some (such as My Last Wish) simply transfer services that have been available in other venues to the web. Others provide visual access to postdeath rituals for those who otherwise would have missed them. Still others create new forms of memorializing the dead. Will these uses of technology greatly transform our experiences of death and bereavement? I doubt it. While the existence of elaborate Life Stories may give us more details about the dead, it is unlikely that they will provide more profound insights than those presented in a good condolence letter. And while observing a funeral online allows the absent bereaved to share some experiences with those who are physically present, an online funeral is no substitute for the real thing; virtual mourners miss the sense of community provided by small talk, hugs, and the time spent together grieving.

Bereavement support

For the bereaved, one of the most important web resources may be access to a community of other bereaved individuals (see Roberts, in press). In some cases, that community is composed of people who experienced the same loss. [...] For example, WidowNet (2004) has e-mail forums, chat rooms, and message boards for those who have lost a spouse, and AARP Webplace (2004) has a general Grief and Loss message board. GriefNet (2004), which is run by a clinical psychologist and mental health volunteers, has forty-seven e-mail support groups, by type of loss and age of the bereaved. Although little research on such online bereavement support groups exists, it is likely that they are beneficial. Hollander (2001), in the only published report of its kind, found that online bereavement support groups provide a valuable community for suicide survivors. Studies of other types of online support groups have found that they foster a sense of community in their members, have many similarities to in-person support groups, and may encourage people to participate and express thoughts and feelings (e.g. Dunham et al., 1998; Kummervold et al., 2002; Winzelberg, 1997).

Thus, the web offers opportunities to increase support in bereavement, at sites that are specifically designed for that purpose, sites that memorialize the dead, and general gathering places.

[...]

References

AARP Webplace [Online]. 2004. "Coping with Grief and Loss." http://www.aarp.org/griefandloss/home.html.

The Body [Online]. 2004. http://www.thebody.com.

de Vries, B., and Rutherford, J. In press. "Memorializing Loved Ones on the World Wide Web." *Omega: The Journal of Death and Dying.*

Doka, K. J. 1989. "Disenfranchised Grief." In K. J. Doka, ed., *Disenfranchised Grief: Recognizing Hidden Sorrow.* Lexington, Mass.: Lexington Books.

Dunham, P. J., et al. 1998. "Computer-Mediated Social Support: Single Young Mothers as a Model System." *American Journal of Community Psychology* 26(2): 281–306.

Forever Network [Online]. 2004. http://www.forevernetwork.com.

FuneralNet [Online]. 2004. http://funeralnet.com/.

GriefNet [Online]. 2004. http://www.rivendell.org/.

Hollander, E. M. 2001. "Cyber Community in the Valley of the Shadow of Death." *Journal of Loss and Trauma* 6: 135–46.

Kummervold, P. E., et al. 2002. "Social Support in a Wired World." *Nordic Journal of Psychiatry* 56: 59–65.

Moss, M. S., Moss, S. Z., and Hansson, R. O. 2001. "Bereavement and Old Age." In M. S. Stroebe, et al., eds, *Handbook of Bereavement Research.* Washingdon, D.C.: American Psychologial Association.

My Last Wish [Online]. 2004. http://www.mylastwish.com/.

Roberts, P. 1999. "Tangible Sorrow, Virtual Tributes: Cemeteries in Cyberspace." In B. de Vries, ed., *End of Life Issues: Interdisciplinary and Multidisciplinary Perspectives.* New York: Springer.

Roberts, P., and Vidal, L. 2000. "Perpetual Care in Cyberspace: A Portrait of Web Memorials." *Omega: The Journal of Death and Dying* 40 (4): 521–45.

Roberts, P., et al. 2000. "A Little Sad, a Lot Stronger: The Impact of Web Memorialization on Bereaved Parents and Others." Paper presented at the Annual Meetings of the Gerontological Society of America, Washington, D.C.

Roberts, P., et al. 2003. "Something More Than a Flat Stone: The Function of Web Memorials to the Bereaved." Paper presented at the Annual Meetings of the Gerontological Society of America, San Diego, Calif.

Roberts, P. In press. "The Living and the Dead: Community in the Virtual Cemetery." *Omega: The Journal of Death and Dying.*

WidowNet [Online]. 2004. http://www.fortnet.org/widownet/.

Winzelberg, A. 1997. "The Analysis of an Electronic Support Group for Individuals with Eating Disorders." *Computers in Human Behavior* 13(3): 393–407.

34
Winston's Wish: For Young People

Forum: My Mother Died*

Jo **posted 31 Oct 2005 20:08**

Hey, My mum died on 22nd Febuary 2004, when i was 14 and everyone told me it would get easier but it hasn't. I love her so much and i try to think what she would tell me to do when i have a problem. It is just so hard. Everywhere you go there is soemthing that i wish she could be here to share with me, and lookign to teh future there are so many things i won't be able to share with her. Everywhere people are sayign how we only get one mum, and it is so true no one will ever have that special bond and it;s gone and i don't know what to do because it's not getting any easier. Everyone on here is so strong. I wish i could turn teh clock back! I wish i coudl talk to my mum one more time, and tell her i love her! i wish things were differnt! I wish it didn't have to happenen to my mum ! I wish life was fairer – so she was still here, with me ! I wish my mum could share all the new thigns with me and be there when i relaly need her! I wish you were here! I wish i coukld change the world! But most of all mum i wish that wherever you are, floting on the clouds?, liivng in the earth or having tea with teh angles ? I wish that you are happy and that i make you proud ! Plz rite back if u have ne thign to saylove Jo xxxxx ((Mum ur my hero!!!))

Helena **posted 25 Jan 2006 15:58**

heya ☺ i no wen u loose ur mum it seems like shes gone for good and thats it but trust me shes stil around you watching over you seeing and sharing everything you do and is very proud of you and loves you very much … in time you will notice things hapening and moving around or things dissapering and you will know its your mum its happened to me from sweets and photos vanishing to my plectrum bein pout in my guitar how she used to have hers lipstik bein smeared down the wall which was obv by her cos it wudnt be moe or my dad and my mum even spoke to my dad on the 3rd year anoversary of her deth she said to my dad tell lenny i like the hair im not to impressed with the lip ring and ill always be watching over her nd takeher to macdonaldsa after college … tat made me so happy … i stil say gd nght to her and tel her i love her … maby it takes a few years for spirits to settle in and be able to show u their stil around but your mum will always be with you !!! xxx im her if u need to talk

---

* All the names have been changed.

Excerpts from Winston's Wish: For young people http://winstonswish.org.uk/foryoungpeople/say/ reproduced with permission.

Sarah **posted 17 Feb 2006 21:32**

hey,! i feel exactly the same as you at the moment, my mum died in july last year and im finding it so hard. i just wish things were different just like you

---

Paul **posted 25 Feb 2006 12:48**

hey its me, Paul i saw ur reply to my topic so i went and had a look at urs and i know exactly how u feel my mum died when i wos 14. im 15 now and i would hav thought it would havs gotten a bit better but i still find myself thinking of her a lot it still makes me sad. so i just want u 2 know that ur not alone and if u want to go out and enjoy urself then u can, dont feel gulty as long as u dont go over the top, i remember the last time i went out and had an amazing time but i got a bit carried away and it made my dad angry i don't know what i woz thinking.

Jo **posted 25 Feb 2006 15:26**

hey Sarah – i'm 16 how old are you ? i know it;s really hard but we have to stay strong together if u need to talk ever i'll be here for u !!! hugs! xx

---

Charlotte **posted 16 Mar 2006 16:39**

Hey Jo i am 11 now how old are you my mum died of cansa brain tuima she was in kirkwood hospice for a little while then she died in her sleep ** huggs ** from Charlotte

---

Jo **posted 5 Aug 2006 20:49**

everyone just remember ur not alone in this – and we will all get through it. at the otehr side we will be so much stronger people – our mums will be so proud

---

Erin **posted 22 Aug 2006 20:28**

hi Jo ... thx 4 ur peply 2 my post (i'm totally lost) it has helped ... i guess ur rite we cant bring our mums back but we just have 2 get on with life! anyway i just want 2 say thank you 4 the reply!

Amy **posted 24 Jan 2007 18:01☺**

message: heya im 14 to my mum died when i was 9 its hard isnt it i h8 it so much no one else realises ... thats why we have each other i understand totally xxx Amy xxx plz write bac to me we cud chat or sumthin

---

Jo **posted 25 Jan 2007 18:49**

hey people try to undertsna dbut its really hard for outr friends becoz they literally have no idea what is like to loose their mums and they never will until it happen to them – which i hope is a long long time away, i wouldn't wish it on my worst enemy. but they do try and it's hard for them as well. I hate it when my friends complain about their parents but it's natural for them and so i just try to keep quite. i hope you are feeling better soon! xx

---

35
Bereavement UK: The Garden of Tranquillity

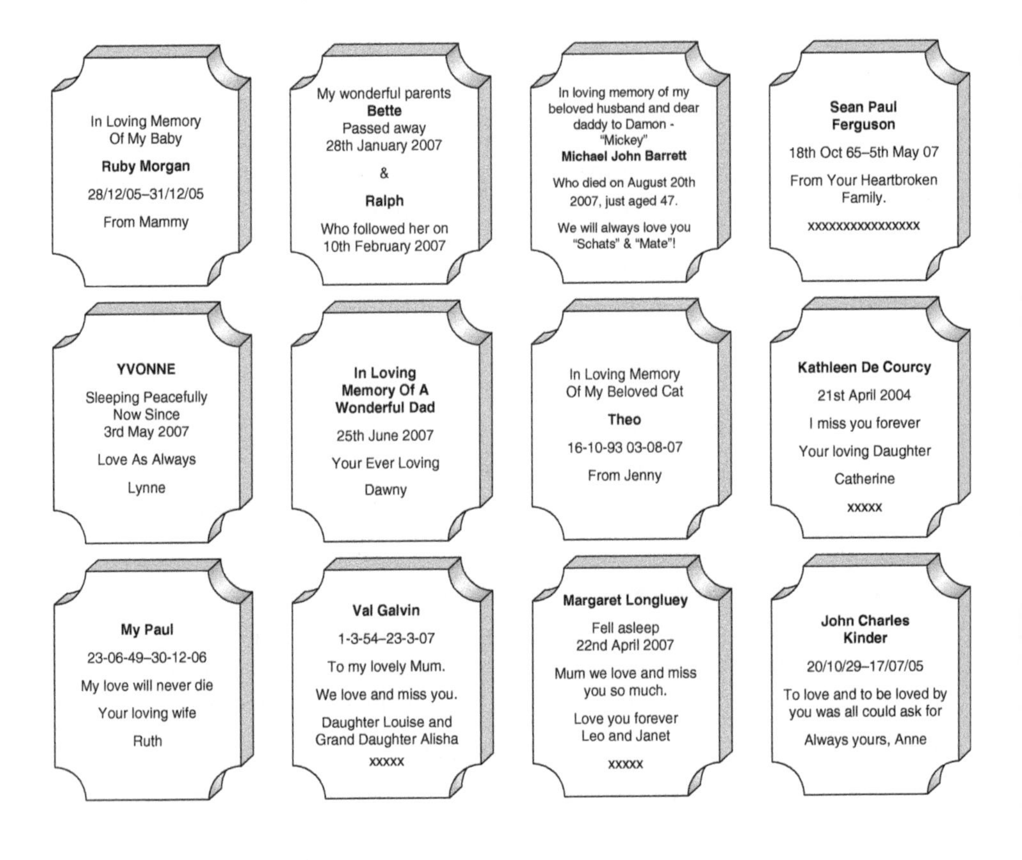

Excerpts from Bereavement UK: The garden of tranquillity http://bereavementuk.co.uk/tranqui.htm reproduced with permission.

36
Andrea Rouen's Farewell

Andrea's body finally gave up on her during the night between 22nd and 23rd May 2007. Those of us who knew her and had contact with her are missing her greatly.

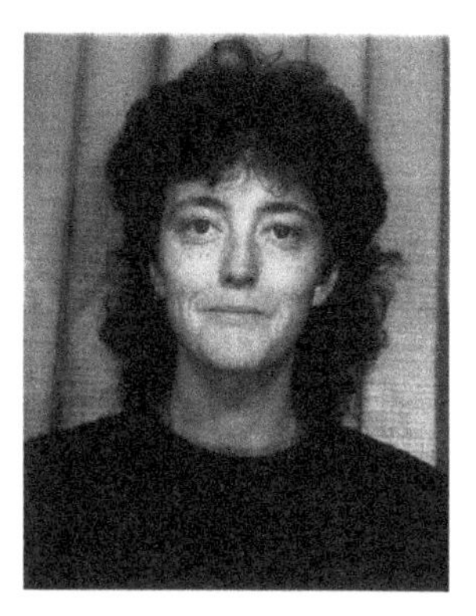

Andrea worked with animals, fostering waifs and strays and rescuing wildlife and dogs. Suffering disability, hearing loss and polyarthralgia causing pain and swelling in joints, Andrea turned to the Internet for communication and the Open University for study.

She was active online within OUSA [Open University Students Association], socialising and providing support for her fellow students. In 2006 she was a member of the Disabled Students Group committee until worsening health forced her to resign. She helped campaign for improved provision for students with disabilities. She was also a major force behind activating the Exeter branch of OUSA.

Andrea's funeral was held on 20th June 2007 at Torquay Crematorium. The funeral was well attended by Andrea's family and friends and many who could not be there sent flowers. Her dog, Badger, was also present. Among the flowers at the back are ones from individual students and from OUSA office.

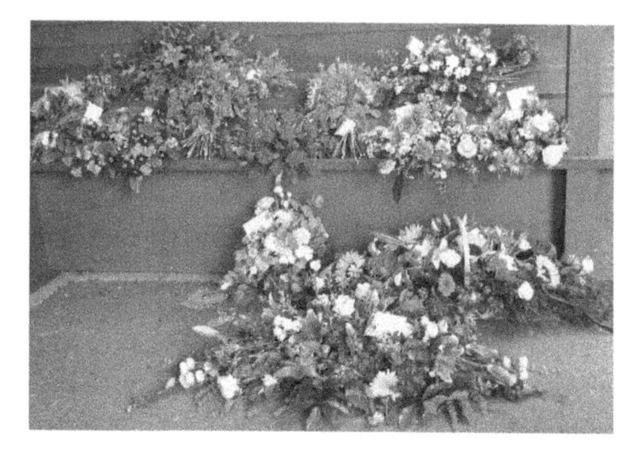

Text excerpts and images from Andrea Rouen's farewell http://ousasw.org.uk/andrea.html reproduced by kind permission of Roz Evans, Kate Graham, Diana Isserlis. 'The Dash' © Linda Ellis 1996 (www.lindaellis.net).

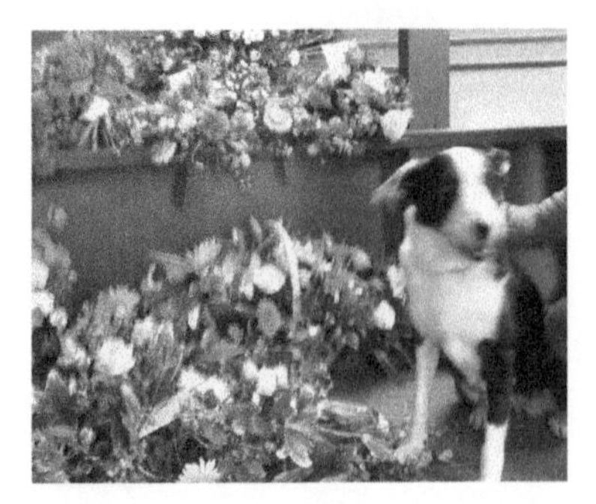

Here is Badger with the flowers. As the helping dog Andrea trained herself, she was her most loyal friend. Badger was Andrea's 'ears', letting her know when there was someone at the door.

The bouquet of flowers at the front is from OUSA Cancer Support, the one on the right with the sunflowers is from OUSA Dogs, and the one on the left is from members of the South West Regional Forum.

Kate's impressions of the day

The funeral was planned in accordance with Andrea's wishes, with her family's full support, and was far from conventional. The cardboard coffin was covered and surrounded by bright flowers including many contributed by Andrea's fellow students.

The funeral director who led the service was sympathetic and professional and helped to ensure that the occasion was memorable for its celebration of Andrea's life and sorrow at its too-early end. The service consisted of readings of poems, personal recollections of Andrea, music and a pagan farewell.

The most moving statement was read out on behalf of Andrea's mother and described her strong character and sense of humour as well as a mother's loss. The descriptions of Andrea's unique character by her close family were strikingly similar to the Andrea we know through First Class [conferencing tool].

Roz Evans spoke on behalf of OU students and explained just why Andrea was so popular in the First Class community. She added that many of those who were not able to attend were marking the occasion in their own way, with candles being lit.

At the end of the service messages were written on or attached to the cardboard coffin as a way of saying goodbye. These included pictures drawn by children in the family. There was also a booklet of personal messages from about 60 students, including the President of OUSA, who all knew her through First Class. A copy of the booklet was also given to Andrea's mother.

There was comfort in confirming that Andrea had been well looked after in her last few weeks, had passed away quietly in her sleep and had appreciated the many messages of support to her during her illness.

Kate

Roz's impressions of the day

I arrived early at the crematorium having allowed for delays, bad weather etc. which didn't happen. Those going to Andrea's funeral were immediately apparent from their bright clothes – including a multi-coloured striped waistcoat – and the fact that small children were playing with a black and white collie called Badger. Kate Graham met me there and we were warmly welcomed by the family.

It was the most original and inspiring funeral I have ever attended. At the beginning we were asked to go and look at the flowers on the casket at the front of the chapel to the music of 'Teach Your Children Well' by Crosby, Stills and Nash and I placed a booklet containing over 60 message from her First Class friends on the coffin. We were handed a simple order of service, with a couple of photos of Andrea and a beautiful poem.

Claire – the funeral arranger – gave a beautiful reading about the need to grieve and how to remember the good times, which brought both tears and laughter, and then Andrea's brother Martin read the poem 'The Dash', which I have attached. A poem by Andrea's sister, Sarah, was then read, followed by a recording of 'What a Wonderful World' by Louis Armstrong.

Lorraine, Andrea's cousin, then read an extremely touching poem which was followed by a message from Andrea's Mum, Dawn, read by Claire – it was the first funeral service I have been to that included a reference to Terry Pratchet and large cabbages! This was both heart-breakingly sad and wonderfully funny, leaving most of us in tears. I had the privilege to be able to follow this with thanks from her 'cyber buddies' for her support, laughter, guidance and wonderful one-liners which were ever succinct and to the point. I mentioned the candles that were being lit at that time and I am sure that your thoughts were with us. We were invited to write messages or draw pictures on the coffin and then a pagan blessing was read – the words of which escape me, but I remember that it summed up the occassion and the person perfectly.

'Time to Say Goodbye' by Katherine Jenkins was then played – which reduced us all to tears once more. Badger seemed to go from person to person saying a personal thank you, and we then moved outside to look at the flowers and reflect.

It is obvious to both Kate and myself that the Andrea we knew from First Class was the same person that those attending the funeral knew – what you saw was what you got. The flowers were wonderful – I had left a bunch from Vivien's garden outside before the funeral, in the place reserved for Andrea; when we got outside again they were surrounded by many other flowers, including those from the Cancer Support Conference, Dogs Conference, The South West Regional Forum and from OUSA in Milton Keynes – no stuffy wreaths, just arrangements, bunches and sprays of wonderful flowers. We had asked permission to photograph the flowers. While we were all looking at the flowers a pair of swallows were flying in and out of the roof above us and sat on the rafter looking at us. Claire commented that as the casket was being put in the car, they left the door open and when they came back there was a bird, sitting on the casket, inside the car – how symbolic!

Kate and I declined the invitation to go to the wake, thinking it best to leave that to her family and friends, and instead took ourselves off to Babbacombe, where we walked along the beach with an ice cream and talked about the service and the wonderful people we had met.

My thoughts are with Andrea's family and friends, including the two lovely ladies who looked after Andrea at home for many months. I am sure that the funeral was as Andrea would have wanted – unconventional and memorable, exactly like the person herself.

Roz

The Dash

I read of a man who stood to speak
At the funeral of a friend

He referred to the dates on her tombstone
From the beginning to the end

He noted that first came her date of birth
And spoke the following date with tears
But he said what mattered most of all
Was the dash between those years
(1962–2007)

For that dash represents all the time
That she spent alive on earth
And now only those who loved her
Know what that little line is worth

For it matters not, how much we own
The cars … the house … the cash
What matters is how we live and love
And how we spend our dash

So think about this long and hard …
Are there things you'd like to change?
For you never know how much time is left
That can still be rearranged

If we could just slow down enough
To consider what's true and real
And always try to understand
The way other people feel
And be less quick to anger
And show appreciation more
And love the people in our lives
Like we've never loved before

If we treat each other with respect
And more often wear a smile
Remembering that this special dash
Might only last a little while

So when your eulogy's being read
With your life's actions to rehash …
Would you be proud of the things they say
About how you spent your dash?

From my dash to yours
Live well, love much, laugh often
Yesterday is history
Tomorrow is a mystery
Today is a present

Linda Ellis © 1996 (www.lindaellis.net)

37
Cancergiggles

Cass Brown

It seemed like a good time to start something new. The news from the meds is pretty crap but hey ho, movement increasingly difficult, some pains are frequent and I know that some of them will last as long as I do. Why then are things funnier than ever before? Why am I relaxed? Happier? More content? What's really weird is that it isn't even slightly drug induced as in the past (not that kind – the necessary ones). Why start writing a blog about a pretty depressing subject? Maybe just one person will read it and take just a little comfort from the fact that it doesn't have to be scary; it does not have to be the end till the The End. Even then maybe there's an epilogue …

A bit of history

OK so maybe I'm just dumb, you know, too thick to understand? Quick history. Diagnosed colon cancer 2000 (I think – but it's not an important date). Stayed pretty laid-back and wondered when the brain would start to get frazzled by the seriousness of it all. Maybe this is an important tip. Total, complete and absolute honesty with everyone about the cancer, the treatment – everything. I have reached the conclusion that most people screw up at this point. Small secrets and untruths (you know – lies) put everyone on the defensive and make them extremely uncomfortable. Funny thing is that if you show people the respect of being honest with them, they respond by being open with you. Even at this early stage, my best mate was asking me to sort out his PC because he didn't want to leave it until it was too late. It lightened the conversation but I knew the bastard meant it.

Ask a lot of questions

As it happened, we did all this crap in a foreign language. I distinctly remember telling my consultant that the only things I was frightened of were things I didn't understand. I didn't understand him because he was speaking French. Actually that's untrue. Because he could see I wanted to understand, he was brilliant. Took loads of time to explain options and likely outcomes (surgery, chemo, radio, operations, death etc.) and every time I saw him (and this applies to every doctor since) I left in a happier mood – even when the news was worsening, grim, bad or downright shitty. I have heard many people protest that if they had cancer, they wouldn't want to know. This is really really, dumb. Have you ever had a nightmare about something real? For almost everybody, the

---

Excerpts from 'Cancergiggles' by Cass Brown www.cancergiggles.blog-city.com/live_with_cancer_1.htm reproduced by kind permission of Kim Brown.

answer is NO. It is the unknown, the shadowy stuff, that normally causes fear. Human beings are actually pretty good at handling real situations, and you will probably surprise yourself.

Family

OK so you handle what is happening to your body. It ain't doing what it should and it's not looking like a picnic from here on in. So you feel sorry for your situation, you regret your wasted life and you sink into a depression. Don't you dare, you selfish bastard! The only people who deserve any pity are those poor souls who will take care of you and watch helplessly as you eventually begin to slide. There's no need to think that you should just accept it all and give up hope. On the other hand, accepting that this could be God's way of telling you that you're not his favourite bunny can actually be quite positive. Odds are that like me, you may get a pleasant, if possible only temporary surprise.

The tests

After a few weeks came the numerous tests. Just about every -oscopy and scan known to man. Take note because this bit is really important! IT DOESN'T HURT! Saw loads of people frightened of what was about to happen to them because it is the unknown. My natural disposition to cross bridges just as they collapse underneath me helped loads. Each time I was pleasantly surprised. Slight discomfort was the worst that happened, but please, please, leave your dignity at the door. Nurses and doctors have almost certainly seen far worse, more ridiculous, fatter, uglier, more ungainly creatures than you. It's not fair to expect them to act surprised when they examine your body. It's like a guy in the body shop screaming or laughing because you've got a dent in the front wing of your Volvo. They see it all day, every day. Give them a break. The only embarrassing thing is BEING EMBARRASSED!

Radio and chemo

So the docs announce that to make you feel better, you are going to be nuked. For good measure they intend to fill you full of some seriously nasty chemicals which you are going to volunteer to carry around with you in a little bottle which will be attached to you via a tube. To make it easy they will put a plug in your chest with a tube which goes up to your head so the chemo can be with you 24/7. Oh and would you mind doing it for, say, 5 months? It doesn't get much better than that. Now here where is there's a real doozy of a question. Do you accept their very attractive offer or not? Hmm. Hair may fall out, bits may fall off, you'll be dead tired and sleep all the time plus you may get a bit ratty. But surely there must be a down side? Yep, you'll probably lose a load of weight. No brainer! Now wait for this. No bits fell off. Often felt pretty tired but not enough to stop me from going to my local bar/restaurant, using the Internet and generally enjoying life. My 'Borg implant' as my daughter calls it (the place where the chemo is delivered into my system) was no problem. Did my hair fall out? I started to go grey about 30 years ago, but after 3 months my wife suddenly started laughing and eventually told me I looked like Mr Spock. My hair had gone thick and turned almost jet black! No doubt you will find it impossible to believe that someone with such a sunny disposition as mine could become irritable. Strangely enough my wife disagreed. Perhaps just a couple of times I …

I just remembered something really funny. Having had my chemo pump for a couple of days (most people don't have these, apparently), I woke up to find that in my sleep I had caught the tube and it had become disconnected. Even my basic physics confirmed that it was likely that the red stuff on the sheets was the liquid that was supposed to stay inside my body and not come out through the tube. I was a tad concerned at this because I know you only have a limited amount of this stuff and it's quite important that you hang on to quite a lot of it. The telephone advice from the hospital was to clean and reconnect it (implying, you dumbo – of course it's not normal). No panic, just pop in when you have a minute and we'll have a look. Moral of this little bit is to forget everything you have seen on TV. When you get used to all sorts of different bits of kit attached to your body they lose their mystique. I can't bleed my central heating boiler but I sure as hell know how to regulate a drip.

Please sit down ...

Doctor says very slowly and gravely 'I'm sorry, you don't have long to live. You only have about er ten ...' Quickly the man interrupts and demands 'What? Years, Months, Weeks?' The doctor continues 'Nine ... Eight ... Seven.' I told this joke to my consultant when I could see in his eyes that he wasn't about to tell me I'd won the lottery. I told a similar one in French when I was first diagnosed. This may seem a flippant or even stupid way to deal with a life-threatening situation. If it was bravado or bluster I would agree, however, my personal theory goes like this. The guy in the white coat, on the other side of the desk, gets up several days of the week, knowing he is going to have to tell people that their life will end prematurely. No amount of cash, free stethoscopes or drugs can make that a good way to wake up. He wants to do his best for you; he will use all of his hard-learned skills, so please give the poor sod a break. My experience is that he needs to laugh as much as you. Help him. Enjoy life. All of it. Even the crap. LAUGH! I also found with one consultant (they are often little gods with their minions) that when I wound up this internationally known surgeon about his shaky hands, incompetence and frequent visits to the golf course, it put him and his whole department in an amiable frame of mind. He is a 20-hour a day, 7-day a week guy who is incredibly skilled. He is incredibly also a human being.

Up to the operation

End of 2000 became ill. Started to live in the bathroom and although the decor was rather pleasant it was not done for this alone.

Visit to my doctor, followed 2 hours later by X-ray, followed by doctor 1 hour later, followed by appointment with consultant 2 days later. You may not appreciate them devouring the legs of small frogs but they sure as hell get this right in France. Really nice guy who talked about ganglions and polyps (in French) and lots of other non-cancer-like things. Seemed pretty relieved when I asked him about the bloody great tumour I had seen on the X-ray.

As I mentioned, I then had tests. A lot of tests. And then some more. The probes and cameras inserted into pretty private places were not too bad. It was the camera crews, soundmen and extras I didn't like.

This is a bit out of context but it has been bothering me. WHY THE HELL DO HOSPITAL GOWNS FASTEN AT THE BACK? As you are presumably there because you are not exactly feeling 100%, why do they think you can fasten several tie strings behind your back? I think they must have CCTV in the changing rooms and sit there howling with laughter as a 17-stone steel worker (that's not me – I don't work in steel) struggles to get into a size 8 mini-dress which has 7 unaligned strings to tie. They then struggle to examine/operate on you because most stuff involves working on you from the front. I want an answer.

Diagnosed cancer of the colon. Large tumour which was unfortunately very low and therefore difficult to treat. Proposal was to treat pre-operatively with chemo and radio for several months and then start cutting. This was to involve a temporary colostomy for a few weeks (turned out to be illeostomy for 8 months) while the bits rejoined themselves. My social calendar at the time was looking pretty thin so this didn't seem the sort of party I should miss. I was a tad annoyed because swimming would be out for the summer. The surgeon assured me (and how French is this?) that I would still be able to drink wine. My wife, Kim, tried to put on a brave face but was hit pretty hard, and the rest of my family must have used a Star Trek transporter to get to me so fast. I merrily went on thinking that soon the reality of this would hit me and I wouldn't be able to handle it. This was before I knew about the other me.

Radio and chemo was a breeze, as already discussed. A bit inconvenient because they refused to replace the bottle of 5FU (chemo) with malt whisky on my occasional days off, but there's more than one way to skin a cat.

I must at this point mention my very good friend Colin. I think he was partially responsible for the development of the second me. As I was completely open about everything that was happening, so was he. During this time we discussed and laughed about (often to the absolute horror of his wife, Chris) the ins and outs of cancer, illness, dying and more importantly to him, how he would keep his PC running when I was pushing up daises. My advice to anyone with cancer is to find someone like this. Your close family are so deeply affected on a practical and emotional level that an outside influence (even if like Colin they happen to be close to the Devil Incarnate) is important. If you think you can benefit from my approach to cancer, find someone who makes you laugh. Colin is the funniest man I have ever met.

The cruellest cut

Over 7 hours and 450 stitches and staples was enough to make even me wince. I can't remember much for several days but know I was packed in ice (which Kim had got from the supermarket), sprayed with iced water and had a large powerful fan 2 feet from my head. I do remember seeing my surgeon a few hours after the op and he looked like hell. Sweating, sunken eyes and obviously completely shattered. At least I had the on-demand morphine. Ten days of no food or drink carrying a drip around were not good for me. I get bored and ratty as quickly as Gordon Brown waiting for the Hutton Report, so I guess this is where the other me stepped in. There is no way that I could handle pain and that level of boredom at the same time. In retrospect the answer was simple: give it to someone else. And I did.

Post op to now

Due to some pretty weird post-op problems I decided to spend a while in bed. Five months on permanent morphine and pain killers, eating nothing. Lost over 40 kilos in weight (jealous?) and looked like a stick insect. I do not recommend this. Several times I was within a few hours of being very dead and each time my wife managed to shock, threaten, plead or persuade me back to life. I really knew nothing. I suspect the other me did but kept it quiet. Eventually became stronger and clawed my way back.

Returned to the UK early 2003. Several hernias a bit of a problem, but they have just been fixed.

After a bunch of advanced scans and other tests we found that the original cancer had spread to both lungs (probably), liver and (probably) pelvis. The other me was quite looking forward to having treatments for these niggles because it would have given him a while in the spotlight, however, the advice was that operations were out and chemo/radio would probably (that word again) only be a holding measure. Time? 6/12/18 months maybe, but maybe more. It made a change from probably.

Now this is really decision time. Hang on to life? Try everything and anything to extend it? String it out for as long as possible so that you are able to breathe? I completely understand those who take this course and pondered very long and hard myself. I decided I would pass. I have been offered and accepted the option of a course of chemo which should have few if any side effects and may give me another few months, but that's it. This could well give the wrong impression of my view of life. I love it. Every single minute, good or bad. A joke I heard many years ago sums up my philosophy: 'If you don't drink, smoke and hang around with loose women, you don't live longer – it just seems like it.' It is quality, not quantity that matters. I know that when I go, it will have a devastating effect on my daughter. Whenever it happens. The way I see it is that the less time she has watching me die – the less time before she can start to get over it – the better. She was aware of everything the first time round, but we have made the decision that she now finds out at the last possible moment. We want her to have as many days as possible, happy, normal, with her father. The same applies to my wife Kim. What happens afterwards when I can't help? I believe that I deal with our situation in the best way possible. I have no answers to this bit. It's the only time I cry.

Thanks to

I have been incredibly lucky to have the support of a strong family. Wife, daughter, father, brothers through to almost long-lost cousins. My illness has bought me genuinely closer to all of them. Their help – practical, financial, but most of all emotional – has been inspiring and even healing. Even though we were in different countries, my two brothers were by my side so fast they must have got whiplash from the car's acceleration. Me being me, I laugh and have fun with them all. I'd hate you to think that this is just a mantra – it isn't. I'm the happiest, most content and relaxed 'dying' person on this planet. We're all 'dying' but just some of us on different time frames. I might even confound them all and stick around longer than expected. There is hope, but I don't spent my time hoping (or even hopping, for that matter). I've learnt to dream. Not in the abstract sense, but I have literally learnt to control what I will dream about. I guess most people have had dreams where they can fly. I have probably had these wonderful dreams a couple of times a year throughout my life. Now that I can concentrate on living I can switch it on in any dream I choose (just for the record, I am currently not using any drugs which would account for this, I am not currently in massive pain and I haven't joined the Liberal Democrats). I digress. I am in absolutely no doubt that without my wife I would be dead already. A couple of years ago she cared for me and literally dragged me back to life when everyone, including the doctors, had just about given up hope. Both her and my young daughter had to cope with my complex medical problems, the practical and financial problems of being in the situation in a foreign country and the very strong likelihood that I would die in the very near (sometimes thought to be hours) future. They were just amazing! This goes back to a previous point. If you ever, for one nano second, feel sorry for yourself, just simply be ashamed. Sorry to turn this on its head, but this ISN'T ABOUT YOU. It's about the people you will leave behind, and soon you will have absolutely zero input into the situation. Use whatever time you have to make them happy and for God's sake MAKE THEM LAUGH. If you have devoted your entire life to being a miserable, selfish, mean and entirely unattractive excuse for a human being, knock it off now! If you are bankrupt, don't have a friend in the world and your family has deserted you, get off your ass and make somebody else laugh. You get just one crack at this. You can't die happy if what you leave is a world of shit and grief. If at some stage in the future my name comes up and it elicits a wry smile from someone, that's good. If it makes somebody laugh, you'll hear me jumping on the clouds.

Cass Brown died on 6 January 2007.

38

Dead Bodies on the Internet

Anna Davidsson Bremborg

Photographs of dead bodies on the internet appear in many different settings. The intention of publishing them might be political, informative, scientific, artistic – or provocative. In this article, the discussions about photographs of dead bodies from two very different contexts are analysed and compared. One is from an international disaster, the 2004 Asian Tsunami, where photographs were used for identification. The other is from a personal catastrophe: stillborn and infant deaths. The discussions come from two Swedish parent communities – www.alltforforaldrar.se (*Everything for Parents*) and www.familjeliv.se (*Family Life*) – both fairly large, with more than 200,000 unique visitors a month.

On 26 December 2004, the waves of the tsunami rolled into the beaches of Western Thailand and in a couple of minutes the tourist paradise had turned into a death place. In Thailand half of the 5,395 victims were foreign citizens, with Sweden being the largest foreign group with 543 dead, 1,500 injured and 15,000 in the area (*Sverige och tsunamin*, 2005). This made the tsunami one of the worst and most broadly experienced disasters in Swedish modern history. But it was also unique in that it was the consequence of globalized mass tourism, a situation no national contingency plans had considered.

That the tsunami occurred during the Christmas holiday added to the chaos. To overcome the lack of official information, special home pages and discussion forums very soon opened. Anxiety, anger, frustration, hope, relief and grief were all given exposure in these forums. However, with notice boards giving information, these home pages were also practical tools in the search for missing persons.

In the forum set up for the tsunami at one of the analysed communities (www.alltforforaldrar.se), one of the topics was the identification of the dead persons. The character of the disaster made the identification of the victims very difficult, and after a few days the Thai authorities published photographs of recovered victims on the Internet in the hope of getting help from families and friends. To involve relatives in the identification of the deceased is common in many cultures, but not in Sweden, where the identification has to be done to by a doctor. In the forum, the Thai pages caused enormous discussions. One message serves as example:

> When I came to this page, I was met with something I never could imagine. I thought I would see peacefully dead persons, lying there, easy to recognize for relatives and friends. But it wasn't like that at all. Most of them looked like swollen balls, black and mangled. I don't understand how they can look so terrible in just a few days.
>
> (www.alltforforaldrar.se, 3 January 2005; author's translation)

Discussions about how bodies decompose followed. The analysis reveals the large gap between traditional representations of dead bodies and reality. The representation of death as person lying peacefully in a bed (Bradbury, 1999) is so strong that even after such a tremendous disaster people thought they would find the dead in this manner. Descriptions of what they saw opened further ethical debates about the use of language. Is it acceptable to say that they 'looked like swollen balls', as above, or as another wrote, 'grilled cracked hot dogs'?

Some wanted to visit the page to 'learn about death', but for many visitors the truth was more than they could cope with, and afterwards they wrote warnings and ethical arguments against visiting them. Many refused – openly – to give out the URL when somebody asked for it, and soon it became almost immoral to be connected with these pages. However, people whose family members were missing regarded the pages as a useful tool in their desperate search. In contrast to the lack of information, communication, help and empathy from the Swedish authorities, the photographs represented the attempts of the Thai officials to do something in a desperately chaotic situation. The web pages were not only an instrument for identification, but also a sign of help to people desperate to find their loved ones.[1]

The photographs of the tsunami victims belonged to a unique situation. But photographs of dead persons on the Internet are not unusual, not even on the parental community sites. During recent years, it has become more and more common to post photographs of stillborn babies on these sites, as well as on other home pages.

Memorializing a stillborn baby can be particularly difficult because of the relative lack of memories and tokens of remembrance. It is only in the last fifteen to twenty years that delivery wards have taken photographs, as well as hand and foot prints of the child, and encouraged the parents to hold their dead infant (Rådestad, 1999). But while the purpose of the photographs from the part of the caregivers was intended to help parents' grieving process and understanding of death, the use of such photographs on memorial sites, Internet photo albums and family home pages is quite different. Like parents of living babies, those of stillborn and dead infants want to show their baby to others.

Although these photographs are important for the parents (Säflund, 2003), the movement to the public arena has not been without controversies. An analysis of discussions, as well as photograph policies on the two community sites, reveals their complexity.

One of the communities (www.familjeliv.se) had decided not to accept any photographs of dead children. To clarify this rule, the editor made the following statements:

- They are interpreted as offensive and thus against the membership rules.
- There are many sensitive members.
- It is not always appropriate to publish things of this nature.

(www.familjeliv.se/Forum-5-52/m1818951.html, 7 January 2005; author's translation)

There were over 600 responses to the editor's statement, and not only from parents with stillborn children. One issue was what should be deemed offensive, and who has the right to judge

1 The photographs were also used by a voluntary organization, Tsunami Souls, who by using professional photo software, enlarged details such as tattoos, clothes, necklaces and other personal belongings and posted them on the Internet together with descriptions of the body, to help with the identification. After a few weeks, the Thai authorities closed their photographic site, and the identification work continued through fingerprints, dental examination and DNA analysis.

the photographs. While the editor, on behalf of some members, argued that photographs of dead children were upsetting, the parents of the stillborn declared that the mere sight of a pregnant woman caused them some distress.

Another question concerned the editor's definition of 'sensitive members'. Why should pregnant women be defined as a group of sensitive members, and not the mothers who had lost their children? His use of 'appropriate' was also put into question. Who defines what is appropriate in a community for parents? And, should we always deny that a pregnancy might end with a death? The editor replied that parents of stillborn children should not be so 'pushy', and that wanting to display a photograph was an 'over-reaction'.

It was clear that the photographs, for the parents of the stillborn, did not only have a memorial function, but also served as signs of their parental identity. The editor's use of ethical arguments against the photographs insulted them deeply. Eventually, the discussion ended in a compromise. Photographs of dead infants or stillborn babies can be published, but only behind a barrier, warning the viewer of the 'sensitivity' of the material.

While the photographs caused major problems for the editor, as well as for some visitors to that site, the other community (www.alltforforaldrar.se) chose a different approach. All photographs are subject to a vetting procedure, and there is no censoring of images of stillborn babies. A photograph of a stillborn baby may appear in the member's presentation room, but also in the avatar (the user's icon) every time a message is posted. The parents of the stillborn, from discussions that sometimes come up on the issue, appear to find this procedure to be fair and reasonable. However, this policy places emphasis on the quality of the photographs, which caregivers at the hospital do not always take into consideration.

Conclusions

The analysis has brought attention to several perspectives on photographs of dead bodies on the Internet:

1. The widespread use of the Internet has opened up new ways of communication, and with it new questions and problems. The diverse policies of the community sites discussed show how general netiquette rules, such as 'not being offensive', are interpreted differently.
2. The Internet has facilitated the movements between the private and public spheres. Regarding stillborn babies, photographs that used to belong to the private sphere have become public when published on the Internet. In the case of the tsunami, it was photographs taken by the official authorities that forced their way into the private sphere.
3. There is a huge ignorance of dead bodies. People's thoughts and representations of dead bodies are based on imagination and expectation rather than experience and knowledge. This ignorance might be due to a fear of confronting death, especially during pregnancy which is supposedly a happy experience.
4. The photographs of dead persons in these contexts have multiple functions. They are not only used for identification or confirmation of death, but also as signs of hope, empathy and identity. The photographs are an important means for establishing identities. Moderators, editors or other members of web communities sometimes misunderstand this vital function, and by using ethical arguments against them may inadvertently offend the persons with bonds to the photographs.

References

Bradbury, M. (1999) *Representations of Death: A Social Psychological Perspective.* London: Routledge.

Rådestad, I. (1999) *When a Meeting is also Farewell: Coping with a Stillborn or Neonatal Death.* Hale: Books for Midwives.

Säflund, K. (2003) *An Analysis of Parents' Experience and the Caregiver's Role Following the Birth of a Stillborn Child.* Diss. Stockholm: Karolinska Institutet.

Sverige och tsunamin (2005) Katastrofkommissionens rapport (The Catastrophe Commission Report) SOU 2005:104. Stockholm: Lind.

39
When Kids Seek Help On-Line: Internet Chat Rooms and Suicide

Katja Becker and Martin H. Schmidt

Many youth in conflict are reaching out to the Internet for virtual support and guidance. This is a brief alert about this new risk confronting children with suicide ideations.

In most countries, mortality from suicide is the second or third leading cause of teenage deaths. The incidence of suicide attempts peaks during mid-adolescence. Evidence supporting existence of suicide contagion continues to amass from studies of suicide clusters and media impact. Suicide increases proportionally to the amount, duration, and prominence of media coverage. Imitation effects depend on the model's characteristics and the extent of behavior reinforcement. The impact of suicide stories on subsequent completed suicides appears to be greatest among adolescents (Schmidtke & Schaller, 2000). Media counseling and guidelines for editors can help minimize imitative suicides (AACAP, 2001). The Internet is an increasingly important medium among adolescents and young adults, who use it as a source of information and to communicate (e-mail, forums, and chat rooms).

In 1974 Phillips coined the expression 'Werther effect' to describe the imitation of suicides presented in the media (referring to the 1774 novel *The Sorrows of Young Werther* by J. W. Goethe, blamed at the time for the many young male suicides like the protagonist Werther). More recently, single case reports about "cybersuicides" have been published (Alao et al., 1999; Baume et al., 1997). One of our patients, a 17-year-old female, admitted she had visited suicide web forums to discuss suicidal thoughts and reliable methods (Becker et al., in press). Another 15-year-old female patient reported that the Internet inspired her to commit suicide as a problem-solving strategy.

Suicide information is easily accessible over the web, as are special chat rooms for discussions with like-minded people. Chat room visits are typical of adolescents and young adults, a group at the highest risk for imitative suicidal behavior. However, suicide forums and chat rooms differ in quality. Some advise acutely suicidal persons to seek help. Promotion and announcement of suicide are forbidden. Chat rooms enable anonymous discussion of a taboo topic at any time without deadline pressure. Some people might experience relief, having shared feelings and thoughts. Furthermore, the links of help organizations offer e-mail contact to those seeking help, which is a low-threshold, informal way to contact therapists.

Katja Becker and Martin H. Schmidt, 'When kids seek help on-line: Internet chat rooms and suicide', *Reclaiming Children and Youth*, 13(4), Winter, pp. 229–30. Originally published as a letter to the editor in *Journal of American Academy of Child and Adolescent Psychiatry*, March 2004 issue (43: 3: pp. 245–7). Reprinted by permission of Lippincott Williams & Wilkins.

Other suicide chat rooms, however, place no restrictions on participants, their mean position being that suicide is a deliberate decision. They postulate an antipsychiatric attitude and give clear instructions about methods, locations, and how to write suicide notes. Some also deal in suicide utilities. Webmasters, laymen at therapeutic counseling, are opinion leaders within a chat room. They are responsible for group consensus, often pro-suicide. Other opinions are not tolerated. Internet use diminishes other modes of communications and heightens social withdrawal, causing a rise in psychopathological characteristics. Ambivalence, an often-precarious balance between a chosen life and a chosen death, which is considered common to suicidal attitude, may tip in the direction of death in response to suicide chat rooms. Suicidal adolescent visitors risk losing their doubts and fears about committing suicide. Risk factors include peer pressure to commit suicide and appointments for joint suicides. Furthermore, some chat rooms celebrate chatters who committed suicide. Imitational learning depends on factors of the model and the reaction of the environment. The virtual community ignores factors such as gender, age, and race, and chat partners can be fantasized as ideal models, thus enhancing imitational learning. The Internet may have a more direct influence than the print media on the Werther effect (Baume et al., 1997), but at the moment we only have single case reports and hypotheses. To prove these hypotheses more research is essential.

Though a cybersuicide or interactive Werther effect is still only speculative, practical implications should be discussed. General prohibition of suicide sites is neither practicable nor reasonable. Site owners should know and follow the fundamental media rules of preventing imitation suicide and post no information on suicide locations or methods or their efficiency or availability. Help-group sites and qualified treatment for suicidal youths should be better promoted. Psychiatrists, parents and teachers should take more interest in their patient's/children's Internet consumption and discuss content with them. In a psychiatric exploration, especially of suicidal adolescents and young adults, questions on media and Internet use should be essential. However, the legal options to prevent cybersuicides should be discussed from a national and an international perspective because of the criminal abuse of the Internet communities.

References

American Academy of Child and Adolescent Psychiatry (2001) Practice parameters for the assessment and treatment of children and adolescents with suicidal behaviour. *Journal of American Academy of Child and Adolescent Psychiatry, 40* (suppl 7) S24–S51.

Alao, A. O., Yolles, J. C., & Armenta, W. (1999). Cybersuicide: The Internet and Suicide. *American Journal of Psychiatry, 15*, 1836–1837.

Baume, P., Cantor, C. H., & Rolfe, A. (1997). Cybersuicide: The role of interactive suicide notes on the Internet. *Crisis, 18*, 73–79.

Becker, K., Mayer, M., Nagenborg. M., El-Faddagh, M., & Schmidt, M.H. (in press). Parasuicide Online: Can suicide websites trigger suicidal behaviour in predisposed adolescents? *Nord Journal of Psychiatry.*

Schmidtke, A. & Schaller, S. (2000). The role of mass media in suicide prevention. In K. Hawton & K. van Heeringen (Eds). *The international handbook of suicide and attempted suicide* (pp. 674–697). New York: Wiley.

40
Resources on the World Wide Web

Sarah Earle

This list gives just some of the online resources on death and bereavement available on the World Wide Web.

Babyloss: www.babyloss.com

The Babyloss website provides information and support for anyone affected by the death of a baby during pregnancy, at birth or shortly afterwards. Resources include discussion forums, information leaflets and online dedications.

Bereavement UK: www.bereavementuk.co.uk

This site offers a range of services including a free public message board, membership to a bereavement Yahoo group and online remembrance.

Blue Cross: www.bluecross.org.uk

This animal charity runs the Pet Bereavement Support Service (together with the Society for Companion Animal Studies). The Blue Cross website provides details of their telephone and email befriender service as well as information on pet bereavement (including children's pet bereavement) and online pet memorialisation.

The Child Bereavement Charity: www.childbereavement.org.uk

This charity provide specialised support, information and training to all those affected when a child dies, and when a child is bereaved.

The Child Death Helpline: www.childdeathhelpline.org.uk

This organisation provides support to anyone affected by the death of a child. Their website contains general information (for example, on the registration of a death and the role of the funeral director) as well as links to other online resources.

The Compassionate Friends: www.tcf.org.uk

The Compassionate Friends offers support to all families bereaved after the death of a child or children. The website provides information about the range of services they provide, which include a telephone help-line, group meetings and a list of useful publications.

Cruse Bereavement Care: www.crusebereavementcare.org.uk

This organisation promotes the well-being of bereaved people and seeks to enable them to understand their grief and cope with their loss. This organisation provides support and offers information and advice, as well as education and training services.

Department of Health: www.dh.gov.uk

The Department of Health provides a range of information and online training and development resources for professionals, plus a selection of online publications and other useful links.

Disaster Action: www.disasteraction.org.uk

Disaster Action offers support and guidance to survivors of disasters and people who have been bereaved. In addition to a selection of online leaflets, this organisation provides information and advice to those charged with responding to a disaster.

Lesbian & Gay Bereavement Project (Terence Higgins Trust): www.tht.org.uk

The Terence Higgins Trust contains information on sex, sexuality, HIV and AIDS. Their online AIDS memorial service is part of the Lesbian & Gay Bereavement Project.

National Association of Widows: www.nawidows.org.uk

This offers support and advice by widows for widows (including both women and men). The site provides information on the association's telephone befriending service, as well as an online discussion forum which is available to members only.

RD4U: www.rd4u.org.uk

This organisation is part of Cruse Bereavement Care but is run by young people for young people. It contains information and advice as well as a message board and gallery. This site also has a 'lads only' section, providing a forum specifically for young men.

RoadPeace: www.roadpeace.org

The charity RoadPeace provides support to those bereaved or injured in a road accident. Amongst a range of services, RoadPeace provides an internet memorial and tribute service.

The Stillbirth and Neonatal Death society (SANDS): www.uk-sands.org

SANDS supports anyone affected by the death of a baby. The website has an online discussion forum, a section devoted to 'personal experiences' containing poetry and stories, a selection of publications and links to further online resources.

Support after Murder or Manslaughter: www.samm.org.uk

This organisation provides support to those who have lost a member of their family or close friend as a result of homicide, and seeks to promote good health for people who have been bereaved. The website contains information about its services, which include a helpline.

Survivors of Bereavement by Suicide: www.sobs.admin.care4free.net/index.htm

This is a self-help organisation which seeks to meet the needs of those bereaved by the suicide of a close relative or friend. Amongst other resources, the website contains information, audio and video clips, testimonies and poetry.

WAY Foundation: www.wayfoundation.org.uk

This foundation provides help and support to men and women widowed under the age of 50 years. Information is given about the range of services they provide, which include newsletters, message boards, chat rooms and a free book loan service.

Winston's Wish: www.winstonswish.org.uk

This charity provides support for children who have been bereaved. The site offers information and other services for children, parents/carers, schools and professionals.

Part IV
Caring for People at the End of Life

Introduction

Sarah Earle and Carol Komaromy

Caring for people at the end of life can be both a rewarding role and a challenging one. In this part of the book, attention turns to the experiences of family members and friends who care for people who are dying, as well as to those who are involved in end-of-life care as part of a professional role.

The pieces presented in Part IV focus on the experiences of friends and family. In the first of these, which has been newly commissioned for this volume, Lydia Chant writes about the care her mother received (who had been living with Alzheimer's) before and at the time of her death. The next piece, also newly commissioned, by Mary Twomey explores the ethical dilemmas she faced when she believed that her father was dying. Then, in an edited extract from the book *Precious Lives*, Margaret Forster discusses the deaths of her sister-in-law and father. The juxtaposition of timely and untimely deaths here challenges the notion of 'natural' and 'timely' deaths. Whilst considerable attention is given elsewhere in the literature to the needs and experiences of family carers, the role of friends and neighbours in providing care is often neglected. In an edited extract from a paper previously published in the journal *Mortality*, Elizabeth Young, Clive Seale and Michael Bury report the findings of a study which highlight this important contribution. Again, the assumptions that underpin the idea of what is considered to be 'natural' are challenged.

The remaining pieces of writing presented here are either written by those who care for the dying in a professional capacity, or focus explicitly on the role of carer. The first two of these contributions, by Alun Morgan and an anonymous contributor, both newly commissioned for this volume, explore the role of the hospital porter. In the following selection, Cynda Hylton Rushton focuses on the role of nurses, urging them to consider their own needs, arguing that they too require self-care, in addition to support from the institutions in which they work. In the next contribution, surgeon Atul Gawande considers the medical imperative to 'save lives', arguing that this is not always in the patient's best interests. The piece by Nancy A. Hodgson, Sheila Segal, Maria Weidinger and Mary Beth Linde explore the contributions of the social worker and chaplain during and after death.

The final three contributions in Part IV also focus on the role of professional care-givers, but here the importance of intimacy and relationships at the end of life are highlighted. Debbie Komaromy, a staff nurse working on a children's neurology ward, reflects on the intimate care provided by a dedicated team of healthcare staff to a 10-year-old boy dying from a brain tumour. Next, and drawing on a selection of case studies, Philip Ball discusses the importance of intimacy and relationships in a hospice setting. In the final piece, Tom Heller reflects on the intimate relationship between doctor and patient at the end of life. Drawing on his early experiences as a family doctor, he explores the management of emotions and considers his own 'professional mask'.

41

Alzheimer's: My Mother's Death

Lydia Chant

By the time my mother died at the age of 80, on 5 August 2003, she was already lost to us. She had been in the care home for 5 years, suffering from a cocktail of damages to her brain: atrophy caused by Alzheimer's; vascular damage caused by small strokes to the brain; multi-infarct dementia; severe brain damage caused by her excessive drinking over many years. As one of the nurses in the hospital ward where all this was diagnosed put it, most graphically, 'Your mum's brain is full of holes'.

In the home Mum had become known as Betty-Boo. Her actual name was Betty. But Betty-Boo was a very different person from Betty. Betty-Boo was, according to the care staff, the life and soul of the party. She flirted with the men, danced and sang. The home seemed to take her over, her familiarity with the care staff becoming easier as her relationship with my sister and I diminished. She was treated like a doll, with fancy hairstyles and dressed in clothes she would have hated. As she gradually sank into dementia, communication inevitably deteriorated with us. Somehow it was persistently difficult to treat her as anyone else other than our mother. As long as she recognized us, even fleetingly, we knew where we stood. But suddenly, it seemed, there was a switch of roles. It came about three years after she had moved to the home, when instead of greeting me by my name she called me Mum. 'It's Mum!' she kept saying, gazing at me in wonder. My sister laughed at this, but somehow I couldn't find it funny.

It wasn't until the day she died that we discovered that the care staff had all been under the impression that Mum had been married to a wonderful American airman called Ed, and had had a very long and happy life with him. On further investigation we discovered that she had talked often about Ed, an old friend of the family, and the care staff had made the assumption that he was her husband, and our Dad. Our actual Dad to whom she had been extremely unhappily married until the day he died two years before her diagnosis, was never mentioned. The care staff were as shocked as we were to discover our respective 'truths' about Mum. I felt quite ashamed that we had not been able to communicate Mum's background to the home, and that her history had been re-written in this way, and gone on for so long.

It is difficult to pinpoint when exactly we knew she was dying. At what turned out to be the beginning of her final year she had suffered several falls, once actually breaking her hip. She had been admitted to hospital and my sister and I arrived to see her struggling on a bed in A&E, fighting off the doctor who was shouting to her. He asked us if she was deaf or foreign, and what language she spoke, and was surprised and apologetic when we told him she was suffering from the later stages of Alzheimer's and couldn't speak, something the home had managed not to communicate to the A&E department. Although her hip was patched up, she was unable to respond to physiotherapy, and this marked the beginning of her deterioration.

In the few months before Mum died, our visits became more difficult and fleeting, as by this time she was unable to talk or even recognize us. Her facial expressions had reduced to a tightly closed chewing or an open, vacant, toothless smile. Her mobility was no more than a short painful shuffle. I worried obsessively about her pain, and was assured that they were able to tell the signs. I wasn't so sure. I began to feel more and more helpless and guilt-ridden. How much could I intervene when she had become the home's responsibility? Mum couldn't communicate at all, so it seemed the home had to speak for her. We became just visitors.

There had been a false alarm the week before she died. We only found out on our regular visit that the care staff thought she'd died when she had collapsed in the corridor, but she had been OK. And now I sat with her at the lunch table. I thought she must be well again, if she was up and eating. But she sat with her head bowed, her glazed eyes gazing beyond the untouched plate. I felt she was closing down, and I desperately wanted her to look at me, to acknowledge me, but she didn't, no matter how much I stroked her arm and spoke to her. I looked up and found that all the other residents around the table were looking at me. Maybe they all knew how desperate I was feeling. I kissed her and left. A few days later we got a call to say that she was very poorly and would we be able to come in the next morning. Although it wasn't mentioned, I read 'very poorly' as 'dying'. I couldn't bear to watch her die, but my much pluckier sister said 'I'm going. She was there when I was born and I will be there when she dies!' So I decided to go.

I woke to such a clear blue sunny day, jarring with the notion of death. It seemed strange on the drive to the home; it felt like my sister and I were out for a jaunt, rather than on a journey to watch Mum die. It didn't seem possible that someone who had been as vital as she had been in my childhood – my abiding memory of her – could just stop existing. I dreaded that moment when the whole world turns.

The home, which we had never visited this early in the morning, was a-buzz with domestic activity: washing machines whirring, vacuum cleaners bashing against doors, pans clashing in the kitchen. All this seemed at odds with the sight of my mother lying on her bed, as still as death, her eyes closed and her arms folded across her chest. She had been dressed in a bright pink nylon nightie, one that wasn't her own and she wouldn't have been seen dead in! Her room was large, with a huge bay window through which the sun relentlessly poured. It was hot and stifling, despite the open windows and the curtains three-quarters drawn.

Mum's two closest care workers, Candy and Ellen, had welcomed us. It felt that they were prepared for us, for the death. Everything felt deliberately normal. Death was not mentioned. We were left with Mum. We were brought tea. Other care workers called in to talk to us and tell us how they had loved Mum and how they would miss her. It was at this point that we discovered about Mum's 'happy marriage'. My sister and I cried a lot, and were brought toilet paper when the tissues ran out. We laughed a lot too. Perhaps the occasion distilled our memories into all that really mattered, the good times. Perhaps we were now old enough to understand more about life. My sister had brought with her a bottle of Mum's favourite perfume, Joy, and delicately dabbed some behind Mum's ears and on her wrists. Candy and Ellen came in at fairly regular intervals to check her. There was a rhythm to all this, a gently rocking comforting. We watched the white butterflies dancing outside the window, and heard the daily traffic on the road over the wall. Life carried on.

In the early afternoon, Candy came in accompanied by an elderly man who was sweating profusely in his tweeds. She briefly introduced him to us as the home's local doctor who, she said, had very kindly come to see our mother. He asked us how 'mum' was, as though we'd popped into his surgery with a cut finger. I was furious about his patronising tone and told him I thought she wasn't very well and might be dying. He smiled weakly and listened to her heart and touched her face with the back of his hand. I asked him how long he thought she had. He ruminated and said that these old biddies can take ages, perhaps a few days, even weeks. At this point Candy rushed to the door and held it open for him. He put away his stethoscope and left as she thanked him profusely for coming. My sister and I looked at each other, confused by this surprising news. Within a few moments, Candy returned with Ellen. They took the blanket away from Mum's feet and looked at her ankles. Candy said, 'Your Mum will die in about two hours.' This was the first and only time death was mentioned.

During the next two hours Mum's breathing became gradually more laboured. At no point was she given anything to drink. It was something that had always bothered me during her time in the home, that there never seemed to be water around. Orange squash, yes, and even hot tea, but no access to ordinary water. I always felt Mum was thirsty. But now, it struck me, it didn't matter anymore. Her breathing seemed to be building to a crescendo, or rather it's opposite. Her colour began to change and we felt strongly that her death was near. I fetched Candy and Ellen. My sister sat on Mum's bed and Candy sat beside her and took my sister's hand. Ellen sat on the arm of the armchair I sat in, with her arm round me. Candy leaned close to Mum and said 'Betty-Boo, it's all right, you can let go now', and kissed her. Mum's breathing had become a long rasping sound. Through my tears I called out, almost wanting to call her back, 'Thank you. Thank you for everything you have done for us.' I felt Ellen tighten her grip on me and she whispered in my ear 'It's all right. We do this for everybody'. A splutter of laughter erupted though my sobs as Mum's eyes opened slightly and she exhaled her final long exhausted breath.

Afterwards I thought about that crucial, though surreal, moment of death and misunderstanding, when crying and laughing became horribly confused. Perhaps Mum herself would have found it amusing; I like to think she would, but I felt cheated out of my final words to her, my way of telling her I loved her.

42
Respect for Autonomy: Easier Said than Done

Mary Twomey

Should I tell my father that he was dying? He had been re-admitted to hospital with unexplained symptoms and no-one seemed to understand what was happening to him. It seemed clear to me, however, that he was approaching death even though the medical and nursing staff involved in his care didn't seem to recognise this. The most I could get from the one doctor who was prepared to talk to me was that 'from the end of the bed, things are not looking good'. I can't say exactly how I knew that my father was dying, but I have looked after a lot of dying people during my nursing career. I'd also seen my father's health deteriorate quite rapidly during the preceding two or three months, so I was reasonably sure even though it seemed impossible to be able to discuss this with anyone.

The fact that his imminent death was not recognised by any of the doctors and nurses caring for him caused me a lot of distress. I would dearly have liked to care for my father at home, but that was impossible. The message that my father was getting from the medics was 'we need to find out what's wrong with you', suggesting that once they knew, they would be able to sort it out and his health would be restored. In the light of this, going home made no sense whatsoever. In order to make that decision he would need to be told that there was in fact nothing that could be done to reverse his deteriorating condition, so that he could make a choice about where he wanted to be. It was too much to ask of someone in his position to believe my one small voice rather than the voices of the clinicians who had such faith in finding out what was going on, as if this in itself would provide a cure.

I couldn't talk through with anyone whether or not it was right to tell him that he was dying. It wasn't at all clear that he would have wanted to hear this, even if it had been recognised. He very much loved his life and he didn't want it to end. He had always hated the idea of dying, even though he longed to be free of the pain he had endured for years. Clearly, even working out how much he might want to know would need a careful and consistent approach from those involved in his care. I couldn't even begin to have this discussion with the nursing and medical staff involved. Nor could I suggest to them that perhaps it was inappropriate to subject him to the scans, blood tests and X-rays that they carried out in their relentless pursuit of a diagnosis. When the ward sister expressed her consternation about the fact that he wouldn't drink and I suggested that this was because he was very close to death, she looked at me in sheer incomprehension.

There was also the problem of what to tell friends and relatives. I felt very strongly that my father should agree any information that was communicated about him, but how can you agree to what you don't know? He was very close to a number of his cousins, but none lived close enough to visit and see for themselves what was happening and it seemed only fair to alert them to the seriousness of his condition. In the end, I simply asked him who he wanted me to contact and what he wanted me to say. 'Tell them I'm seriously ill but getting better', he said. A very good friend of mine had offered to do the phoning for me and she was present during this discussion.

'Leave out the "getting better" bit', I said. It was a compromise – he retained a degree of control and I felt that I'd alerted people without deceiving him. But it did mean that I couldn't really talk to him about what was going on. Maybe those important last conversations are a myth anyway. Maybe the end of life is mundane and caught up with practicalities for most people, but even so it would have felt better to have some acknowledgement of what was going on.

The care that my father received wasn't poor care, at least not on this occasion. It was simply inappropriate care, and it was care that precluded any of the discussions we might have wanted to have. It also made it impossible for my father to choose where and how he might want to die. As it was, his death was noisy and distressing and I did finally lose my patience with the doctor who was desperately putting up a diuretic drip because he had no urine output, and the nurse who was desperately trying to apply an oxygen mask and a horrible plastic hypothermia blanket because they were still so locked into treating symptoms even at this late stage, less than an hour before his actual death.

What perhaps made things harder around my father's death was that the same thing had happened with my mother ten years earlier. My mother had been frail and anorexic for years and had developed pneumonia and various other problems, some of which had led to her emergency admission to hospital. Her time in hospital was traumatic and confusing for us all, and my father became ill himself whilst trying to cope with it. When I visited after a short time away, it seemed clear to me that she was extremely ill and I wanted to discuss this with those caring for her. Most importantly, I felt that I should encourage my father to visit despite feeling ill himself, as it seemed to me that she would die quite soon. My attempts to discuss this with the nurses got nowhere and eventually I saw one of the medical staff; this doctor listed my mother's symptoms and told me what they were doing to correct each one. When I suggested that my mother was dying, she looked appalled. I thought that perhaps she simply had a problem with using the words 'dying' and 'death', so I repeated my thoughts and reassured her that I had worked with a lot of dying people. At this point she told me that it wouldn't be worth her doing her job if she just gave up on people, and I realised I was still getting nowhere. And perhaps she was right, perhaps my mother would recover from the overwhelming number of symptoms that were assaulting her, although it still seemed unlikely. Despite my experience, who was I to think I had a better assessment of what was going on? How could I go home and say 'Dad, make a big effort to come and see Mum now, because I think she might be dying', when no-one agreed with me?

My mother died eight hours after my frustrating conversation with the doctor who was caring for her. I should have had the courage of my convictions and encouraged my father to visit, but I didn't. After my mother died I felt extremely angry with the doctor who had failed to see that my mother was so ill and had dismissed my feelings so readily. I felt angry that she was so into listing symptoms and treatments that she couldn't see the impact on the person who was too frail to cope with all of that. And angry that she clearly saw accepting someone's imminent death as 'giving up on them'.

That was ten years before my father's death, but even a decade later, very little seemed to have changed. It felt lonely being the only person who seemed to know what was going on, and it felt impossible to do the things that I thought were right, namely open the door to the possibility of talking about death with both my mother and my father. Both my parents had short illnesses before they died, but these were not unpredictable deaths and I am not clairvoyant. But it was shocking to me, having gained my experience in district nursing and in cancer care, how firmly the doctors and nurses caring for both my parents were locked into symptoms and treatment. They lacked experience and expertise in caring for dying people, but would probably not have recognised this at the time, and it was this that shut down all of my attempts to talk about what was happening on both occasions. How can we hope to promote choice and control in dying when those responsible for delivering care are not able either to recognise, accept or discuss that someone is dying?

43
Precious Lives
Margaret Forster

[…]

This doctor was a youngish woman. That must mean she was particularly brilliant, I thought. Hard enough to qualify as a doctor, doubly hard to have reached such a position in a London teaching hospital. But she certainly did not seem brilliant at establishing a relationship with a patient. She was perfectly pleasant but avoided eye-contact and never once expressed sympathy with Marion. Her attitude seemed offhand, almost flippant. Maybe this was a pose she'd perfected to cope with potentially emotional encounters; maybe she had to behave like that in order to get through these stressful sessions. At any rate, she plunged straight into an account of how the radiotherapy would be administered, talking rapidly and constantly opening and shutting the drawers of the desk, though never revealing what she was looking for. […] She asked if there was anything else we wished to know which she hadn't covered. Anything else? I produced my bit of paper. We hadn't started yet.

[…]

It was bothering Marion at the time that if the nose tumour had been diagnosed as malignant earlier, when she had first been sent to hospital – after complaining to her doctor of that 'something' in her nose – her life might not now, be in danger. She knew perfectly well that blame was irrelevant now, but she wanted to know the truth. She also wanted to know if the initial excavation of the tumour had not gone far enough. The doctor's drawing was to demonstrate the normal depth of tissue removal and then how in Marion's case the malignancy had in fact spread deeper without showing any signs of having done so. 'Unless,' Marion said, quite sharply now, 'the surgeon had gone deeper.' The doctor said that there were no indications that he needed to. It was just bad luck. Marion said she might take this enquiry further. The doctor shrugged. It was up to her. She stood up, making it clear it was time for us to go. Out in the cold street, Marion seethed. She was sure a cover-up was going on. She knew it was tedious and pointless to persist in trying to establish the truth, and that she would waste a lot of emotional energy she could scarcely afford to spare in doing so, but she couldn't give up. It was her life and she wanted to know – even if it made everything worse – whether it had been put in peril through an oversight.

[…]

I hardly dared to mention the word 'hospice'. Hospices were for the dying. If I suggested Marion went into a hospice it would be interpreted as a sentence of death. But I knew hospices were not just for the dying. I knew, through a friend who worked in one, that they were also for respite care for those suffering from cancer. Patients could go in for a couple of weeks and

---

come out again. I rang my friend and asked if there was even the most remote chance that the hospice where she worked in Hampstead, the Marie Curie Centre, would take in Marion so that she could survive the rest of her radiotherapy treatment. She said she was sure there was and would herself set admission procedures in motion if Marion was agreeable. I rehearsed what I was going to say, how I was going to explain the benefits of going back each day from the radiotherapy to a place where people would know how to look after a person in her condition. But I didn't need to recite my lines – both Marion and Frances burst into tears of absolute relief. They had a bag packed in a flash and within twenty-four hours Marion was settled into a room in the hospice with immediate advantage. [...]

[...]

Christmas Day was grim. Annabel and her family came on Boxing Day, as usual, but Marion was too ill to join us. She was in bed most of the time, feeling worse than she had ever felt even though the radiotherapy had ended. New Year was no better, because for the Davies family, being Scottish, it was the big festival of the year and not to be able to celebrate it appropriately was miserable. 'It might be my last, who knows?' Marion said. And what did I reply? That of course it would not be – the same old instinctive reaction of denial, the same refusal to contemplate the possibility of death.

[...]

Another very disturbed night followed, and then, in the morning, Saturday, we had great difficulty keeping Marion in bed once the Marie Curie nurse had gone. She was agitated, incredibly restless, and kept trying to get out of bed, but I couldn't let her until Frances came down. She sat on the edge of the bed, the covers thrown back, and I sat facing her, my knees jammed against hers, talking frantically about Armistice Day ceremonies. When I had to call for Frances – I could no longer prevent Marion from trying to stand – she was calmer, and agreed to stay in bed until the district nurse came. When she appeared, it took the three of us to support Marion. It was only two steps to the chair she would sit in while the bed was made, but it seemed like two hundred, so agonisingly slow were her movements. The bed was quickly remade but then the pressure sore had to be dressed, and that was best done with Marion leaning against the bed while we held her up, so we prepared ourselves for the ordeal (and I thought how easily this could have been done in the hospice).

Getting her onto her feet from the chair hard enough, but the moment she was at last upright, Frances and I on either side and the nurse hovering, she collapsed – swiftly, absolutely suddenly, just *down.* The nurse wanted to send for more help but we wanted to let Marion try to get up first. We sank down beside her and talked quietly to her and stroked her back, and told her to take it easy, not to worry, there was plenty of time, plenty of time ... Her breathing was heavy and we wondered if she had simply fallen asleep, but eventually she sighed and said, 'Wait, wait,' as she always did. And then, as we levered her up, she managed to get onto her knees and, after another long wait, to raise herself further, and we quickly pushed the chair beneath her and lowered her into it. It was easy then to shove the chair towards the bed and half tip her out onto it. The sore was dressed, the neck bandaged and at last she was tucked up, drowsy and still breathing heavily. 'Thank you, now,' she said, and went to sleep, propped up high on her pillows but soon slumping forward.

We were drained and exhausted, and went to sit in the next room, shaken by the drama of it all. The nurse came in. 'This can't go on,' she said: 'Marion needs to be in a hospice.' Frances lashed our, saying she would not accept that the hospice could look after Marion better than we could. The nurse muttered something about a hoist, as she had done before, and a pump to deliver the morphine into the system more effectively, and yet another kind of water mattress. A hoist? Fine, we'd get a hoist, and a pump, and the special mattress: we'd order them all on Monday. The nurse was silent. Then she said that the point she'd warned us about had been reached and that she couldn't accept responsibility for letting this go on. She'd be discussing it with her superior on Monday. We said nothing, still too distressed to argue effectively. We went on sitting there after she'd gone, trying to calm ourselves. Marion's breathing was so very loud we could hear it through the wall. It was laboured and harsh. We went to look at her and saw mucus dribbling from her nose. We had to keep wiping it away, but this did not disturb her. She slept on, and we thought that was good. Perhaps she would sleep all day and make up for her broken night.

Friends and family came and went, tiptoeing up the stairs, talking in whispers. I wasn't scheduled to stay that night – it was to be my first night at home for a week and I was going to try to have a ten-hour sleep to prepare myself for what might be the long haul ahead. A kind friend of Marion's and Frances's was to take my place, and off I went at about five o'clock, reluctant to go but knowing I should be sensible. We all had to husband our resources. I went to look at Marion before I left. There was no change. She was still asleep, as she had been since ten in the morning. She looked awful, all hunched up, nose leaking, face swollen and grey, hair damp with perspiration. I walked home, glad to be outside, though the air was cold and far from fresh all the noisy way until I'd crossed Highgate Hill. I went straight to bed, slept for a few hours, and then woke around three. When the telephone rang just before seven I was ready for it. Even before I answered I knew Marion was dead.

The relief was instant. It was all over, all that horror. She'd died at home, and though only the Marie Curie nurse was with her when her breathing stopped, she had indeed been surrounded by those who love her, as she had wished, right up to her last moments of consciousness.

The dead body was lying flat on its back, covers pulled up to its bandaged neck, hair neatly brushed. Since I'd seen such bodies before, four of them by then, I had no fear of this one. A dead body was an object, a cadaver, no longer a person, and I'd always found it strangely reassuring that this should be so. Before I saw my first dead body, a cousin's, when I was fourteen or so, my imagination had terrified me – I'd envisaged something repellent and disgusting, something hideously disfigured, perhaps covered in slime, or crawling already with maggots. The reality had surprised me. I felt nothing, confronted with the corpse, which had seemed bloodless and devoid of any ability to scare. But I'd wondered if I'd feel differently when the dead person meant something more to me. If corpses had been loved when alive, would they have the power to be frightening or at least to awe? I found they didn't. […]

Some people want to see the body, some don't, saying they prefer to remember the person alive. Some invest the corpse with feeling and treat it as an object worthy of reverence or even as a still living, but sleeping, thing. Either way, dead bodies have their own mystique and a house with one in it can make people shudder. Frances wanted Marion's body to be seen and could herself scarcely bear to leave its side. She maintained that Marion looked peaceful and that she had a smile on her face. To me, her face looked grotesque, distorted by the cancer cells packed within it, her smile – a grimace. I looked at it and banished it, replacing it with Marion's face before the disease began. For me this lifeless thing, lying there, had nothing to do with Marion. But for Frances, it did. She didn't want to part with Marion's body and wouldn't let it be taken to a funeral parlour, not yet. She was desperate to keep it, to invest it with continuing meaning.

[…]

The day Marion died, 12 November, I didn't write my usual weekly letter to my father. My sister telephoned him and told him the news and he said, 'Pity,' as expected. But I wrote the following week, touching only briefly on the funeral and otherwise concentrating on family chitchat, as I knew he would want me to do. And I resumed the regular telephone calls, taking up my place again in the rota. This seemed to please him very much – 'Grand,' he said, 'back to normal now.'

[…]

In February, it was my turn to go for a short visit [...] We left him fairly cheerful that particular afternoon, and the next time we came he wanted to go out. But from then on we were never certain how we would find him. His favourite carer was concerned. 'He isn't himself,' she said. She thought he might be sickening for something. I could hardly restrain myself from suggesting 'Death?' On Friday 23 July, we visited but he wouldn't go out. We passed the time well enough with me showing him photographs of Carr's biscuit works at the turn of the century which I'd been collecting for a book I was researching. He liked that. It stimulated him to talk about Carr's and my aunt who worked there. On Sunday, when I made my daily phone call, there was no answer. The telephone was right beside him, on the little cabinet next to the chair, from which he could not now move unaided. I rang the nurses' desk. Arthur, they told me, had elected to stay in bed all day. He didn't want to be bothered with the telephone. They'd rung to warn me and to assure me he wasn't ill, just tired, but there had been no answer. [...] They said not to worry, they'd report his condition in the morning, which they did. [...]

The doctor came again the next day and this time I was there to see him. He said he'd like a word with me. A nurse showed us into the little staff-room so that we could have some privacy. The doctor explained that my father's chest infection was a form of pneumonia. One of his lungs was already quite heavily infected and the other slightly. He was wondering how the family felt about this. His language was so careful I in turn wondered if he was using euphemisms, but I don't think he was. It then emerged that, apart from the chest infection, there was something else wrong which would need admission to hospital for proper diagnosis. (The home didn't have the necessary sophisticated equipment.) At least this was easy to respond to. I said my father emphatically did not want even to go back into hospital and that he'd said so, loudly and often: he was not going into 'that place' again. So that was clear. The doctor nodded. There was still the delicate matter of antibiotics. A course of these might clear the infection up. There was a pause, perhaps unintentional, and he asked once more how the family felt about this. I said we were all in agreement: we wanted our father made comfortable and relieved of pain if possible, but that was all. 'He says his life is no fun now,' I said. The doctor smiled sympathetically. He said my father had amazing power of recuperation, but he was nearly ninety-six and very frail and anything might happen, quite suddenly, antibiotics or not. I said I understood.

What I thought I understood correctly was that my father was literally at death's door at last, arriving by a different route from Marion but finally there. I wanted him now to go through that door as smoothly as possible, with no banging on it, no standing in the rain waiting, with none of the hanging about he loathed. He looked so peaceful already, lying still like a good boy, pyjamas buttoned up to his neck, white hair neatly brushed, muscles of his face relaxed. He was ready. He could just drift into death. No more hauling him about, no more bruising of his poor limbs with every assistance give, no more forlorn hours trapped in his chair. I wished I had said, 'Please, no antibiotics.' But I didn't want him to be in pain and a chest infection is painful. It was a Catch 22 situation: deny him antibiotics and he might suffer unnecessarily. If he didn't respond, that was different. And I doubt if the doctor would have permitted me to insist on antibiotics being completely withheld.

[...]

[...] I realised my father had shrunk in the last few weeks. His head wasn't anywhere near the head-rest. He had withered away to such an extent that it looked like a child's body curled up there. He looked like a rag doll, merely a bundle of clothes, limp and loose. I realized he could hardly see out of the windows – he had sunk so low in his seat – and I longed to pull him upright. [...] What defeated me was why we, meaning the society in which we live and by whose rules and laws we are governed, allow no escape for people like my father whose life had gone on so long that its quality was eroded to the point where it was no longer precious, either to him or to those who cared about him. It was wearing and wearying, this agonizing, long-drawn-out descent into death. [...]

I was not at home when the matron tried to reach me on 11 December, so she rang Pauline and told her our father was 'really poorly'. Pauline correctly interpreted this as dying and left immediately to go to him. She rang me from his bedside that evening and said that it was impossible to assess the situation yet. [...] Would he rally, as he always had done? Would the antibiotics once more have a miraculous effect? [...] The next day, Pauline rang to say that our father seemed brighter. He was still in bed and his breathing was laboured, but he was talking and objecting to various things she was doing in mistaken efforts to please him. [...]

Pauline was there to give me a daily report throughout the following week. She began to realise that 'really poorly' did mean dying this time, but that still no one could estimate how long it would take. Could be weeks, even months. Or could be days, even hours. [...] I knew the night shift ended at seven o'clock and that this was the best time to ring, when the nurses did the handover in their little room. The nurse who answered was silent when I said I was coming and would she tell my father. 'I'm so sorry,' she said, 'but your Dad passed on about two o'clock this morning.' They'd rung Pauline to tell her and she hadn't rung me, I imagined, because she saw no point in waking me up then.

I rang her at once. We both agreed we felt absurdly shocked – absurdly, because this death had been expected for so long. Expected and wanted. But still we were shocked and disbelieving. He *couldn't* be dead at last; it seemed impossible that this torment had ceased for him. Then there was the regret that one of us had not been with him, actually there holding his hand (if we'd dared). Pauline would've stayed all night if she had known the end was so near, but nobody had predicted that death would come quite so soon. It didn't really matter, of course, since he was said to have died in his sleep, as Marion had done, and Pauline had been with him when he went to sleep – there if not at the literal end then at the end of consciousness. [...]

My father's death was the end of a long, long tough march, but I didn't seem able to rest. I was still on that arduous march with him, still going through the motions of keeping him company. It was as though, because he was so very old, he had come to seem immortal. I had despaired of death for him. The grim reaper had kept passing him over, constantly rejecting him, and I'd lost faith in him even being chosen. It would never be his turn – and then it was, and the shock was all the greater for being deferred.

I thought the relief I looked for might wash over me once I'd seen him dead. Maybe I didn't really believe, on one level, that he was. Maybe I needed to see his dead body to be convinced this was not a trick. [...]

These have been two stories not of life but of dying. They have been about two people for whom life was precious in quite different ways and who approached death with quite different attitudes. Both died bravely, in that neither made those around them suffer. They had no self-pity and made it as easy as possible for their loved once to witness their decline. One, my sister-in-law Marion, was, in effect, given the means to end her own life whenever she chose. She could have overdosed on liquid morphine and shortened the time she had left. But she did not choose to do so. Under no circumstances would euthanasia have been acceptable either to her or to anyone involved with her. If she wanted to go on living no matter what state she was in, then we wanted it too. She made her choice and it was absolutely respected. But my father was never given the choice. He was the one who had come finally to regard his own life as no longer in the least valuable. He was tired of it. But he was obliged to go on. There was to be no cutting short of his dying, inevitable though it had become. It is as though we take a pride in seeing how long we can prolong a life which is clearly over.

It seems odd. It seems wrong.

44

'It's not Like Family Going, is it?'

Elizabeth Young, Clive Seale and Michael Bury

Introduction

Research into the care provided for dying people and for those bereaved has tended to emphasize the needs of family and professional carers over those of friends. [...] These two foci have led to the consideration of the needs of palliative care professionals and family members over those of the small but significant group of friends and neighbours who are in caring relationships with dying people.

[...]

There have been limited empirical studies exploring the friendships of those who are dying. It is at this critical time, when people are faced with changing circumstances and possible imminent death that friendships are likely to be highly significant. Yet research has remained focused on family or professional orientations. This [piece] describes the role of friends and neighbours of people who are dying. [...]

Secondary analysis of qualitative data drawn from a retrospective survey of bereavement focusing on the nearest person at the time of death (Cartwright & Seale, 1990) is presented. The main focus of the original study was on services provided for the dying person. The study was based on a random national sample of deaths of people aged 15 and over who died in 10 areas of England. Eighty deaths registered in 1987 were selected in each area, and interviewers visited the home of the person who knew most about the last 12 months of the deceased's life. An 80% response rate was achieved.

[...]

The roles played by friends and neighbours: friendship as kinship?

[...] The boundaries between friendship and kinship may often be unclear, providing the opportunity for friends to act 'as if kin'. Indeed, many of the respondents referred to their relationship with the dying person in kinship terms, particularly when they were describing the depth of the relationship. Comments from several informants make this clear. For example:

> She was like a sister to me.

Elizabeth Young, Clive Seale and Michael Bury, 'It's not like family going, is it? Negotiating friendship boundaries towards the end of life', *Mortality*, 3(1), 1998, Taylor & Francis Ltd, reprinted with the permission of the publisher (Taylor & Francis Ltd, www.informaworld.com).

> My husband was like a relative to him … my husband had lost his own mother and father and Paul used to live next door to my husband, so in a way was like a father to him.

> I miss her badly. I didn't mind looking after her. She was a good woman, like a sister to me.

These comparisons between friends and family were used by the respondents to illustrate the strength of the friendship. The kinship relationship was used as the standard against which comparisons could be made. One close friend expressed it this way:

> We've had some good times and some sad times. I was closer to her than her family.

Another respondent, expressing the ambiguity of many relationships stated:

> Although I was very close, it wasn't an emotional involvement. He could have been my brother.

When discussing grieving, one respondent made it clear that her friendship relationship with the deceased could only be valued in retrospect, after the burden of caring had ceased:

> I've missed her more recently. When she died it was a relief. Now I miss her as a friend.

Another close friend said:

> I feel a little empty at times. We used to do everything together. I felt comfortable. It's like losing a limb. People used to think of us as a team.

Respondents also reported being involved in intimate and arduous caring tasks for the deceased:

> I was washing, cleaning, plus she had a dog. I had to look after the dog as well. I could have done with more help.

> Looking after her was a full-time job. She was over 16 stone. I first became involved ten years ago when her husband sent for me. She was in a terrible state with being doubly incontinent and with four bed sores … I just could not manage her anymore … the nurses who came in were no help they only dressed her legs and left me, *a neighbour*, to deal with the bedsores.

The categorization of friend and neighbour appear to be flexible for respondents. The respondent quoted above for example, defined herself as close friend at the beginning of the interview but referred to herself as a neighbour in this response, signaling a shift in perceived level of responsibility that she felt should be borne by a non-family member. The caring tasks became onerous for other close friends:

> The crux came when she became doubly incontinent and her mind had got to the point where she had forgotten how her body functioned. It was winter, I was changing her clothes three times a day and my self control snapped and I shook her very hard to stop her sitting down without her pants. I was so upset by my behaviour and frightened by what I had done that they agreed to put her in a home.

What is striking about the accounts is that the descriptions are very similar to those provided by caring family members in other studies of informal care. The respondents, when thus involved in caring, were not constructing boundaries to the practical help provided, though they were often aware of them. The most intimate and heavy tasks were being performed as if kin and, as with kin, this could be done either willingly or with a sense of the negative demands it involved.

Some respondents described one of their roles as being the prime decision maker on behalf of the dying person, particularly in relation to the place of care:

> I sometimes wonder whether I should have moved her four years ago, but I think it was right. I was a beneficiary and she said she couldn't cope anymore so I moved her near me.

> It was just that I didn't want him back in a flat on his own. They said he would have to go back until a place in an OAP home was found for him, but I was adamant, and they, the social worker, found him a place ... Now I wonder if I did right. The place they sent him to was such an awful place.

Both of these respondents questioned the decisions they made on behalf of the deceased. The decisions were being reviewed and justified in retrospect. The responsibility associated with this type of decisions making is onerous and, consequently, the decision-making role appeared to be less comfortable for the respondents compared with the practical caring role.

Boundaries to the caring relationship: duties, obligations and rights

The relationships reported in this study all had boundaries which the respondents were attempting to define, even in retrospect. Some described their family relationships as taking precedence over friendship. In particular, family commitments were used as a way of drawing demarcation lines under the caring elements of the friendship. These were especially emphasized by friends/neighbours though not exclusively so:

> I didn't really have to look after her. She was my friend, her family gave her all the help she needed.

> I have to go to work and look after my family and they have to come first.

> I never went in the doctor's surgery with him, I just used to take him. After all, I wasn't family and I had to respect his privacy.

There was also a sense of duty expressed:

> I was always aware of my duty to him, I just couldn't zoom off. I had to make sure he was alright.

> What would you do? – it's a duty you have to do.

> It was duty, but I was only a friend. I used to do things and he would tell me not to. You really can't take over in somebody else's home.

Duty and obligation were used as a way of justifying involvement. There appeared to be less need for justification for being involved in caring tasks than in decision making.

[...]

Reference

Cartwright, A. & Seale, C. (1990). *The natural history of a survey: an account of the methodological issues encountered in a study of life before death.* London: King's Fund.

45

A Fridge too Far?

Alun Morgan

> The Lanesborough, a St. Regis Hotel, captures the grace of the Regency period. Ideally located in elegant Knightsbridge, the residence is minutes away from the exclusive shopping of Harrods and Sloane Street.*

This quote from The Lanesborough website, which includes photos of sumptuous guest rooms and views looking out onto London's Hyde Park Corner, feels a million miles away from my work as a porter at the Old St George's hospital. But The Lanesborough, reputed to be the most expensive hotel in London and where every room has a private butler, and the Old St George's Hospital, are in fact one and the same place.

In the early 1970s as a student in London, I took at holiday job as a hospital porter at St George's. The building was constructed as a purpose-built 350-bed hospital between 1827 and 1844, and at the time of my working there still retained what seemed to me a darkly authentic old-world feel. It was a bit like the ghosts of Florence Nightingale, George III, Queen Victoria and Charles Dickens had all been rolled-up into one, and were very much still around. A porter's pay in comparison to a student grant was very good money. But I was only vaguely aware when I started that one of my responsibilities as a porter was to collect the bodies of patients who had died and transport them from their beds to the basement mortuary, where I would put them in a giant fridge.

I'm not squeamish. Well, I thought I wasn't. I'd worked previously in another hospital as a ward-orderly, in a holiday job from school, but I'd never seen a dead body before, let alone a fridge full. To say that I was initially freaked-out by the experience would not be entirely true. I was VERY freaked-out!

The porters' room was pretty uncomfortable; a rather smelly and smoky den by the main side-entrance. The supervising porter would receive phone calls from the wards and from other hospital departments and porters would be allocated to the various tasks in rotation. When each task had been completed, such as wheeling a patient from the ward to X-ray, or from outpatients to the ward, or delivering blood samples, the porters would return to their room. By this random process, on average, each porter would probably receive a request for a mortuary trip about once or twice a week.

So, how was it actually done? Well, there's a special trolley. This is probably why you are unlikely to have seen bodies in winding-sheets being shuffled around your local hospital. The

---

*Lanesborough Hotel:
www.starwoodhotels.com/stregis/property/overview/index.html?propertyID=1435

trolley is a sort of gurney with a rectangular body-sized tin box on the top. To put the body in, you lift the lid of the hinged-box and when closed, a clean white blanket is placed on the top. All you then see is two porters pushing a rather high trolley with a blanket on it. It's as easy as that – no need to frighten the horses.

Most of the Dickensian wards in St George's had the old-style long lines of beds, with heads against the wall. By the time we arrived on the ward the nurses would already have laid-out the body and wrapped it in a winding-sheet. But the patients would all see us coming with the obviously empty trolley, and I always wondered what went through their minds. I remember feeling that the patients seemed like survivors in a macabre session of hospital Russian-roulette, in which the Doris or Dan in bed number five with whom they had probably been chatting on the previous day, had drawn the short straw and accepted the loaded revolver. I was a young man, in my early twenties. I had grown up in an idyllic country village and in the late-1960s had, to a large extent, identified with the hippie culture. In my naiveté when starting as a porter, I remember feeling extremely surprised to find myself wheeling dead bodies in a tin box in front of a captive audience of bed-bound strangers. It was a bit of a shock to the system, to say the least.

On one such visit a porter colleague, an old-hand and decidedly blasé, paused before we left the ward to check if the deceased patient's identification tag had been attached to her big toe. Unfortunately, this pause was directly in front of and in full view of the line-up of predominantly older bed-bound patients. It is to be hoped that during this full, side-on opening of the box, that the fellow patients of the deceased were not wearing their glasses. I can't remember, but unfortunately I suspect they were though, because all I can recall are the stunned looks on their frozen faces.

There were some things I never got used to, such as lifting obese bodies, especially those with only one leg; or bodies so thin that they were little more than skeletons; or mortuary attendants eating their sandwiches next to the fridges. There is also something very odd about opening one of several fridge doors to be met with the tops of six heads on six bodies, stacked-up. I had taken the porter's job because I'd heard that it was good pay for relatively easy work. I hadn't expected, however, in what to me in advance seemed to be a relatively simple student-oriented income-generating enterprise, to enter an environment where I would confront full-on the menagerie of my unconscious feelings, fears and assumptions about death. At that time, no one to whom I was close had died. I don't think I had avoided thinking about death; I just never really had occasion to. In many ways, of course, I appreciate that I had been very fortunate. But it also meant that I was entirely unprepared.

The hospital, and particularly the mortuary, had for me a darkly Gothic feel. Occasionally I imagined that I was caught up in a murderous Victorian melodrama in which Count Dracula would leap from the shadows at any moment. At other times I would inwardly recoil in horror when dealing with the mortuary staff. How strange it seemed, I thought, for anyone to choose such a career. What did they talk about with their families and their friends? Surely they either had no friends at all, or their only friends were either other mortuary attendants or undertakers? I understood that doctors and nurses dealt directly with death, but their principal aim was to prevent it happening – so perhaps that was OK? I wondered at times if I would have been less jumpy if I had been working in a modern and much more 'clinical' environment devoid of powerful cultural memories of late-night, black-and-white TV spine-chillers?

Sometimes, for patients who had died in accidents, we were asked to take bodies from the mortuary fridge to the Chapel of Rest to be viewed by relatives. These bodies were not in winding-sheets but in vestments for viewing, and so they appeared as real people. This was quite disturbing for me, especially when they were around my age. Come to think of it, I was always much more disturbed to see their faces and thus engage with the identity of the real people, imagining their lives and their families. For me it was always an uncomfortable meeting, with individuals so recently and so strangely no longer there.

St George's Hospital at Hyde Park Corner finally closed its doors in 1980, in preparation for its transformation into The Lanesborough hotel. I suppose the mechanism we used for transporting the bodies from the ground floor to the basement mortuary, a hand-operated lift in which we pulled the trolley down using ropes, has gone now. It's probably been replaced by a sauna or a gym, or perhaps it's the rest area for a horde of personal butlers, a sort of latter-day porters' lodge? Maybe the ghosts of Doris or Dan are still roaming the corridors along with the old Earl of Lanesborough, who had formerly owned the site and who died in 1736? For me, however, my time at St George's was an important rite-of-passage. It is where I developed a much deeper understanding of and respect for death; and, of course, it's where I learned much about life and about myself as well.

46
A Porter's Story

Anonymous

I first met Peter when I started work as a hospital porter. He knew just about everything there was to know about being a porter. I thought he was someone I could learn a lot from, and within a few months we became really good friends. We often worked together and shared many experiences.

I remember particularly a young girl who came into hospital. She was very ill. It was likely that she would die, and her parents knew that. Her father had watched how we remove bodies from the wards around the hospital, and when his daughter passed away he asked if there was a way we could take her to the mortuary without putting her in a mortuary trolley, or 'box'. He had seen the trolleys we use. We have two: one is a long steel box on wheels, the other is like a theatre trolley except it has a canvas cover which goes over. Neither is very attractive, and a lot of people get quite upset when they see them. It is obvious what they are for. Once, we were bringing a body down in the lift. A lady was rushing to the lift and called for us to wait. We tried to ignore her but she put her hand on the door to stop it closing and came into the lift with us. When she saw the box she shrieked and jumped out of the lift.

We gave the father's request some thought. Peter had an idea to put the young girl's body on a patient's trolley covered up to the neck with a sheet and an oxygen mask on her face with oxygen running. We could then push her around corridors and it would look as if she was sleeping. No one would know that she was dead. It would look as if we were taking her to another department for treatment.

No one objected to the plan. The ward sister was very helpful. Her concern was for the other children on the ward. She didn't want them to see the dead girl, but she agreed because she thought they would be even more curious if they saw the steel box. The worrying part for us was getting her past other children, but we managed to get all the nurses to agree to keep the children in their rooms.

So we took the girl to the mortuary on a trolley. We didn't have to do the job, but both Peter and I felt that it would be easier for us than the other porters as we were more mature – some of the others were very young. That is the only time I have ever taken a child's body from the ward. It is not a common occurrence. I've taken more babies to the mortuary, but with babies it is simpler. It's just a little box – people don't know what you are carrying.

The girl's father came with us. He held her hand and talked to her all the way. I can't remember anything he said. It was his private moment and not for us to pry. When we got to the mortuary he came in with us. Normally it's against the rules to allow anyone in, but we bent the rules that day. He wanted to see where she was. She was put into the refrigeration unit and he was there when that happened. It must have been upsetting for him, but we had to wait for the funeral director and bodies need to be kept cool.

The media image of a mortuary with long filing drawers to store the bodies is quite old-fashioned. If you have a separate drawer for each body you need to refrigerate every drawer individually. In our mortuary the refrigeration unit has 18 doors, 9 at either side. When you open a door there are 4 racks for storing bodies. It's just like a big fridge. If you open one door you can see lots of bodies. The reason there are doors on both sides is that the pathology lab is next door. If a post mortem is needed, they can take a body out from the other side where the lab is.

When the girl's father left, both Peter and I were very emotional. We had tried to keep a tight rein on our emotions and not show them to the father, not because we wanted to appear cold but because we felt it was unprofessional. It was unspoken at the time, but when we talked afterwards we agreed that the grief we felt was nothing to do with the family and they should be protected from it. We were both very reflective and Peter was desperate for a cigarette, so we went to one of our usual smoking places and talked while Peter smoked. He empathized with the girl's father about the mortuary trolleys. He said 'I don't want to go in that box either'. He said to me that if anything were to happen to him in hospital, he would like to be taken to the mortuary in a bed instead of a box.

Several months later I arrived at work one morning to find my supervisor waiting for me. He told me there was a problem and that he needed to talk to me somewhere quiet. When we got into his office he told me that we'd 'lost Peter'. I didn't know what he meant. I said, "What do you mean, has he left?" Then he told me that Peter had died. I asked when this was and he replied that it had only been an hour ago – Peter had been at work. He had come to work on his scooter. It was a cold December morning and, when he arrived, Peter said that he wasn't going to do any work until he'd had cup of tea and a cigarette. He spent some time chatting to a nurse in the smoking room and when she left he was on his own for about 5 minutes. A colleague went in and called to him to ask if he wanted another cup of tea but realised that Peter was very still. He was sitting, but had slumped forward a bit. They called for the crash team but they couldn't save him. At the time they thought he had had a heart attack, but later found out that it was an aneurism: nobody could have saved him. It was a very peaceful way to die really. He wasn't in any pain, which is a comfort I suppose.

Before I arrived at work, Peter's body had been moved to a private room. He was left there all morning for us to go and pay our respects if we wanted to. When I went into the room to see him I said, 'Why have you done this to me, mate? It's not on really. You can't leave me on my own with these young idiots.' I told him that I loved him and that I'd miss him.

I did Peter's work that day. I volunteered. I thought, 'I'll do this for Peter'.

Later, when I was talking to my colleagues, I recalled the conversation Peter and I had only a few months earlier when he said he didn't want to go to the mortuary in a 'box'. One of the managers remembered having a similar conversation with him. It was agreed that we would honour his wishes and take him to the mortuary on a bed. We would give him an oxygen mask with oxygen running, the way that he had suggested for the young girl. We wanted to avoid parading him up and down corridors, but it was quite a long way from the ward to the mortuary. We decided to clear the basement corridor and take him via the lift to the basement. That way there was little chance of members of the public seeing him. It was a well-organised operation. Someone called the lift and held it so members of the public were kept out.

I wanted to be one of the people who took Peter to the mortuary. There were four of us, me and his supervisors and manager, which was good. When it came to putting Peter onto the rack in the fridge, I just couldn't do it. I got very upset and I was sent home.

Peter's funeral is a bit of blur to me really. I don't really go for the religious side of it – the songs and prayers. His coffin was draped in his Spurs black-and-white scarf, and one of his step-children wore a Spurs scarf in his honour. When we went for the burial I wanted to be closer. The other porters all stood back and said that I shouldn't go closer, but I did.

I went to see Peter's grave lots of times. It's a funny thing. I'm not religious, but standing at his grave I feel as if I have a connection with him.

47

Caregiver Suffering is a Dimension of End-of-Life Care

Cynda Hylton Rushton

Caring for dying people is one of the most challenging and rewarding dimensions of nursing practice. For most, the rewards of being a skillful partner on the journey toward death overshadow the impact on themselves. Caring for the sick and dying requires a kind of service that either nurtures or depletes caregivers. To truly care for another means that nurses suffer for and with their patients and families. They are attuned to the whole person and are skillful in identifying sources of physical, emotional, spiritual and social suffering. Nurses respond to the suffering of dying people through their presence, skill and compassionate action. But there are times when suffering for and with another causes conflict, distress and disintegration of the person.

Suffering defined

Reich describes suffering as "an anguish experienced as a threat to our composure, our integrity, and the fulfillment of our intentions, and more deeply as a frustration to the concrete meaning that we have found in our personal experience. It is the anguish over the injury or the threat of injury to the self and thus to the meaning of the self that is at the core of suffering." This definition offers insight into the responses of nurses who experience anguish and distress as they attempt to provide compassionate care to dying people. Who they are and how they see themselves as a person and as a professional can be threatened on many levels. For example, value conflicts, competing obligations, moral distress, inter-and intra-professional disrespect and institutional constraints can cause nurses to suffer and can erode their integrity.

Responses to suffering

Ideally suffering for and with our patients invites compassionate responses by nurses. Compassion allows our hearts to be open and enables us to use our skillful means for the benefit of the patient and their family. If nurses are to respond with compassion to the needs of patients, they and others must first recognize their own suffering. Manifestations of suffering include physical, emotional, behavioral, and spiritual dimensions. [...]

Cynda Hylton-Rushton, 'Caregiver suffering is a dimension of end-of-life care', reprinted with permission from *The American Nurse*, November/December 2001, published by the American Nurses Association.

What to do about our suffering?

Acknowledging our suffering, naming it, giving voice to it and bearing witness to it are important steps toward creating an environment of integrity. Many nurses will need help in naming and articulating the nature of their suffering. Educational sessions that include experiential exercises are a first step in sensitizing nurses to the issue. Forums such as psychosocial or ethics rounds, staff support sessions or debriefings after a patient dies can also create a supportive space for sharing, reflection and resolution. A mental health professional or other skillful practitioner can facilitate such sessions.

Initially, nurses will need assistance to address the physical, emotional, and behavioral responses to their suffering. Once these reponses are addressed, interventions aimed at addressing the spiritual dimensions of suffering can be instituted. Techniques, such as meditation, yoga, bodywork, image work, creative arts and music may be useful. Opportunities to become acquainted with these techniques and to incorporate them into the practice environment can offer nurses important tools to enhance their resiliency and minimize the detrimental effects of suffering.

Creating a culture of self-care is another important dimension of addressing caregiver suffering. The newly revised *ANA Code of Ethics for Nurses With Interpretive Statements* includes a plank that says, "The nurse owes the same duties to self as to others, including the responsibility to preserve integrity and safety, to maintain competence and to continue personal and professional growth." This professional mandate invites us to consider ways to transform our professional norms to honor values of wholeness, appropriate boundaries, self-respect and integrity. Nurses themselves must take the initiative to develop new professional accountabilities.

Nurses also must partner with the institutions where they practice to create a practice environment that is grounded in integrity. With the nursing shortage escalating, institutions must consider the impact of caregiver suffering on the workforce. Denial of its existence and failure to respond to the legitimate suffering of nurses will further erode the profession. As a profession, nurses must unite to advocate for practice models that celebrate and respect the contributions of nurses and nurture their physical, emotional, and spiritual well-being.

Suffering for and with our patients will always be a dimension of nursing practice. Our challenge is how to care for ourselves so that we can continue to care for others.

48
Always Fight

Atul Gawande

The seemingly easiest and most sensible rule for a doctor to follow is: always fight. Always look for what more you could do. I am sympathetic to this rule. It gives us our best chance of avoiding the worst error of all – giving up on someone we could have helped.

However, it doesn't take long to realise that the rule is neither viable nor humane. All doctors have patients they are unable to heal, or even to diagnose, no matter how hard they try.

I was walking down the hallway one day when Jeanne, one of the intensive care unit nurses, stopped me, visibly angry. 'What is it with you doctors?' she said. 'Don't you ever know when to stop?'

That day she had been caring for a man with lung cancer. He had had one of his lungs removed and had been in intensive care for all but three weeks of the five months since. A pneumonia that blossomed in his remaining lung early after surgery had left him unable to breathe without a tracheotomy and a respirator. He had to be heavily sedated or his oxygen levels dropped. He received nutrition through a surgically placed gastric tube. Sepsis claimed his kidneys and the team put him on continuous dialysis.

It had long ago become apparent that a life outside the hospital was not possible for this man, but neither the doctors nor his wife seemed capable of confronting this truth – because he did not have a terminal disease (his cancer had been removed successfully) and he was only in his fifties. So there he lay, with no evident hope of progress and his doctors simply trying to keep him from falling back.

As we talked, Jeanne also told me of doctors she thought had stopped pushing too soon. So I asked what she felt the best doctors did. She thought for a while before answering. Good doctors, she finally said, understand one key thing: 'This is not about them. It's about the patient.' The good doctors didn't always get the answers right, she said. Sometimes they still pushed too long or not long enough, but at least they stopped to wonder, to reconsider the path they were on. They asked colleagues for another perspective. They set aside their egos.

This insight is wiser and harder to grasp that it might seem. When someone has come to you for your expertise and your expertise has failed, what do you have left? You have only your character to fall back upon, and sometimes it's only your pride that comes through. You may simply deny that more can't be done. You may become angry. You may blame the person – 'She didn't follow my instructions!' You may dread just seeing that person again. I have done all these things. They never come to any good.

In the end, no guidelines can tell us what we have power over and what we don't. In the face of uncertainty, wisdom is to err on the side of pushing, to not give up. But you have to be ready to recognise when pushing is only ego. You have to be ready to recognise when the pushing can turn to harm.

In a way our task is to 'always fight', but our fight is not always to do more. It is to do right by our patients, even though what is right is not always clear.

49
The Social Worker and Chaplain During and After a Death

Nancy A. Hodgson, Sheila Segal, Maria Weidinger and Mary Beth Linde

[...]

The social worker

[...] As the family moves from hope for recovery to anticipatory grief, the social worker offers encouragement and support to help the family be there for the person who is dying. The social worker matches the level of involvement to the needs of each family member who has made a decision to be there for the dying process. Matching resources to financial, social, emotional, or legal concerns for families can also provide the family with the emotional reserves to be there for the dying person. Providing the family with information and education regarding options and next steps in logical, nonmedical language can help demystify the treatment and care plan. Information, updates, and guidance in making decisions can return some sense of control.

Any family member's decision to be present through the dying process cannot be taken lightly or for granted (Byock, 2002). Emotional strength, poise, and insight into this transitional stage of life are required. Important discussions with family members often concern the situations that prevent the family from being emotionally present. Family relationships or past experiences may make it difficult as family members fight the reality of the situation.

Listening with your mind and your heart is key to being there when caring for the family members of dying patients. Family members may be unable to articulate concerns about their inability to be physically present for the suffering and dying because of, say, unresolved conflicts, another family member's illness, or financial or job pressures. In situations where geographical distance prevents families from being there, the social worker may be the supportive link, helping family members to feel more connected to the dying person and to each other.

The case of Rose. When Rose's son. Steven, got the call that his mother's condition was deteriorating, he was a six-hour plane ride away. A new job in Detroit kept him from making frequent trips. The social worker arranged nightly phone calls with the son so that he could communicate concerns to the healthcare team and connect with his mother while she had the strength to speak. The regular, predictable contact provided Rose with the reassurance of Steve's ongoing involvement in her care. As Rose's condition worsened. Steve relied on the social worker to provide detailed information and to let him know when he needed to get on a plane. In this

---

Nancy A. Hodgson, Sheila Segal, Maria Weidinger, and Mary Beth Linde, 'Being there: Contributions of the nurse, social worker and chaplain during and after a death', reprinted with permission from *Generations*, Summer 2004, 28(2): pp. 47–52.

situation, the social worker honored Steve's wishes and helped him moderate his guilt at not being present until the final moments of Rose's life. Rose seemed to be waiting for Steve's touch and permission for her journey.

After the death. The social worker helped Steve to gather Rose's treasures and listened to flashes of Rose's life as each memento was packed. They shared stories of Rose's recent life before the decline – Rose's love of Bingo, Rose zooming around the hallways in her electric chair, her love of music and entertainment and expressing herself creatively with her hands in art classes. This interaction gave Steve a balance to what he witnessed at the end and what had come before.

Whether the social worker attends the funeral or memorial service depends upon the depth of the relationship with the person or the family. The decision or attend Rose's funeral was an easy one – Steve personally asked the social worker to be there. After attending Rose's funeral service, the social worker and the chaplain at the facility where Rose had lived planned a memorial service there that Steve, staff, care-givers, and residents could attend before Steve left for his home.

The social worker initiated phone and e-mail conversations with Steve until Steve was ready to let go. After a short while, shorter conversations and longer time between call-backs or responses to e-mails were signals that he was ready to move on, and the social worker became a part of the past for Steve.

The chaplain

The essence of the chaplain's role is to be fully present in relation to the emotional and spiritual realities of life's crises and passages. For the chaplain, being there means offering the gift of 'spiritual accompaniment' to individuals and families 'in whatever they are experiencing, wherever they are' (Friedman, 2001). To this awesome and humbling task, the chaplain ideally brings a heart open to the vulnerability, sorrow, and sanctity of being human. As the chaplain listens with reverence and gently reflects on the feeling that are present, those facing death may experience the relief of being completely heard, understood, and honored. Assured of the chaplain's being there, in the midst of the pain and the fear, patients and family members may feel safe to express their thoughts and feelings – no matter how difficult or seemingly unacceptable. Thus they may open themselves to meaningful communication and, for the family, the beginning of healthy grieving.

The case of Marsha. Such was the spiritual journey made by Marsha, whose once robust 87-year-old father, Iry, was losing his appetite and his ability to swallow. Marsha clung to the idea that if she brought him some favorite foods be might eat more and 'recover his strength.' Her daily visits were always at mealtime, and each day she brought to the nursing home 'something that Dad used to love.' Wanting to please his daughter, Iry took as much as he could get down, but he coughed through each bite and frequently experienced intestinal pain. The staff was concerned about his discomfort and about Marsha's pattern of denial.

One day, after she had established an empathic connection with Iry's daughter, the chaplain was able to gently reflect Marsha's feelings and help her open up to the reality of losing her father. 'I know how much you love and cherish your father and that it gives both of you pleasure when you bring him some of his favorite foods, but what's happening to him isn't really about the food,' the chaplain said. 'What the team is saying is that he's eating less and less because his body seems to be shutting down.'

'I know it will only be a few more weeks,' Marsha responded somberly, after a pause, 'but I feel like I can't go through this again. It's not even two years since I lost my husband.' Marsha's tears began to well, and she soon gave in to the reality of her grief and allowed them to flow. She had not been with her husband at his death – he was on a business trip when his heart attack struck – and she could only imagine the horror of his last minutes. This is what death meant to her: a merciless, tragic wresting of a life that left her feeling stricken and powerless.

After allowing as much time as Marsha needed to express he sorrow and helplessness about her husband's death, the chaplain suggested that her father's death might be different. For one thing, it was not untimely but rather marked the completion of a long and full life. Most important, knowing that his death was imminent, Marsha was provided with the opportunity to say good-bye.

For the next two weeks Marsha's visits were no longer focused on food. She was able to be with her father for hours at a stretch, sharing memories, expressing gratitude, and sitting quietly by his beside. On the last day of Iry's life, when Marsha expressed concern about his increased suffering, the chaplain asked if Marsha thought she could tell him that he didn't have to keep struggling, that he could just rest. Soon after, Marsha saw the tension leave his body, and she was by his side when he took his last breath.

After the death. Three weeks later Marsha expressed gratitude to the chaplain for helping her to find the strength to be there and 'to say the things that were too difficult to say. ... It changed my whole attitude to death,' she stated, 'It was, well, it was beautiful.'

The presence of a chaplain at this stage – whether in the elder's home, the hospital, or in a long-term-care setting – can have the powerful effect of fostering or reviving the spiritual connections that provide comfort and support to the dying person and her loved ones. Those who know that a chaplain will see them through the funeral, burial, and early stages of mourning find immense relief from the anxiety of having to face it all alone.

Even those who have ongoing affiliations with a church or synagogue may seek the continued involvement of the chaplain who has 'been there' for the dying process. This is especially true in long-term care, where over time the chaplain may have become the elder's rabbi or pastor. However, it usually is in the best interest of the deceased's family to rely on their own clergy and congregation at this time, for it is they who will be the family's most important source of support going forward. Chaplains who decline to officiate at the funeral service can still provide continuity of spiritual care to mourners by initiating the contact for funeral arrangements, by agreeing to deliver a prayer or a few reflections at the funeral service, by simply attending the service, or by making a condolence call after the funeral has taken place.

Chaplains in long-term care can also provide grief support by convening a memorial service in the facility where the individual resided at the time of death. Gatherings such as this also serve two other grieving constituencies who usually do not have the opportunity to attend a funeral: the staff who cared for the individual and the other residents who shared her life.

[...]

References

Byock, I. 2002. The Meaning and Value of Death. *Journal of Palliative Medicine* 5(2): 279–88.

Friedman, D. A., ed. 2001. *Jewish Pastoral Care: A Practical Handbook from Traditional and Contemporary Sources*. Woodstock, Vt.: Jewish Lights Publishing.

50

The Intimacy of End-of-Life Care

Debbie Komaromy

Ollie was a 10-year-old boy whom I met while working as a senior staff nurse on a children's neurology ward. As with all the families I have met and cared for while their child is dying, I have never forgotten the time I spent with Ollie and his family. However, the time with Ollie, his family and the team I worked with have stood out as exceptional. Ollie himself was an incredibly caring and empathic child, and his mother's extremely vulnerable position meant we also felt intuitively protective of her. The bond that our team built, both between us as nurses and between Ollie's mother and us, felt unusually close. On reflection, it feels that we wanted to take care of both her and Ollie, and protect them from the heartbreaking emotional journey that they were on.

Ollie's mother was 34 weeks pregnant when we first met them. Ollie's father had left the family home relatively recently, leaving Ollie as the sole male in the household – a role he took very seriously. He would constantly pay attention to his mother's needs and was always concerned about her. He was particularly devoted to ensuring that his mum's pregnancy was going well and was excited about the prospect of a new sister. Ollie and his mum clearly supported each other and had become a close-knit family unit. However, he was still a boy who enjoyed having lots of friends and worshipped his local football team.

Ollie first came to our ward for investigations into seizures which had started very suddenly. He had also been having some early morning headaches and episodes of vomiting. Immediately we knew that things would probably not be good for Ollie, as these are classic signs of a childhood brain tumour. Unfortunately, our suspicions were confirmed and a very large, and probably fast-growing, brain tumour was found.

After breaking this difficult news to Ollie's mother and then to Ollie, he was immediately transferred to a children's neurosurgical unit so that as much as possible of the tumour could be removed. This was a difficult time for our staff as we had developed a strong relationship with both Ollie and his mum. When we handed their care over to another team, we felt a sense of needing to make sure they would be okay; there was an instinctive protective mechanism that the whole team felt. The bond of trust that had developed between us and Ollie and his mum felt strong. We had worked hard to earn it – to make sure we always told Ollie and his mum the truth, and protected him from painful experiences when we could. We didn't want to let them down – or for another healthcare team to let them down. We felt they were so alone – it was Ollie and his mum against the world, against all the things that life was currently throwing at them, and we wanted to be able to help protect them against something, even if it was just making sure that the new ward knew exactly how he liked to be told things or what made him smile when he was having a bad day. With Ollie's mum being so heavily pregnant, she also appeared physically vulnerable, making us feel as if we should help to protect Ollie's unborn sister too.

We were also realistic enough to know that we may not see Ollie again, so there was a sense of potential loss too.

Ollie came back to us a few days later and started radiotherapy and medications to try to shrink the remaining tumour. We were aware that he had an extremely aggressive form of cancer, and that Ollie would be unlikely to survive. During this time Ollie continued to be concerned about his mum's well-being, rather than his own. He would tell jokes and funny stories to his mum and the nurses, and we began to see that Ollie had a character larger than life. There was also an increased amount of physical contact between Ollie and his mum; more hugs and cuddles – even though at times he would become embarrassed by them, particularly if there were any men around to witness them!

A few days later Ollie rapidly deteriorated and began having continuous seizures. It was clear that there was serious swelling occurring in his brain and that the treatment may not be working. Ollie recovered from this episode sufficiently to regain consciousness, but now had difficulty moving around and had become dependant upon his mum and our team for his physical care needs.

We nursed Ollie through this period with a very small team of nurses. Generally there were only five nurses who cared for him throughout his stay, and we were all close as a team. Many of us had worked there for a number of years and had developed strong friendships working together. Each day and night we would ensure that one of us was on duty to care for Ollie and his mum. We looked to each other for support during this time, and sharing the care between this small group of nurses led to a strong support network between us. We would spend time together discussing how we would care for them, and let each other know how things were going, keeping in contact on our days off. Very frequently we would just all meet for a drink after work, to talk things through before we went home. It felt as though we all knew that we had someone we could turn to in the team, to help share the difficult moments. Our medical team, particularly the junior doctors who were there every day with Ollie, also got to know Ollie and his mum well, and eventually it felt that there was an intimate team caring for this family.

Over the next few days Ollie gradually deteriorated. As he was no longer able to move from his bed, his mum had taken to lying next to him and holding him for long periods. Physically this was very difficult, as she was now heavily pregnant. During one of these times they talked about his expected baby sister. Ollie had thought of a name for her, and asked his mum if she would give her this name from him.

It was clear to both his mum and our team that Ollie knew he would not survive for much longer. Shortly after this, Ollie became unconscious. His mum continued to hold him for as much of the time as she could, but it was becoming more and more physically difficult as Ollie was almost as large as her and now immobile.

We started to spend hours with Ollie's mum, sitting in the room with both of them, talking about his life and listening to her thoughts and fears. Much of these intimate discussions happened in the early hours of the morning, when these were no other visitors and she could not sleep. During these times we would also discuss what would be likely to happen when Ollie died – the physical aspects of his death, and what she wanted to happen after this time. We also focused more on caring for her physical needs: trying to make sure we provided food and drinks for her; sitting with Ollie whilst she had a shower or slept. She would worry that he might die without her being awake, so we made sure one of us was always there with her and Ollie. She didn't want to miss her final goodbye.

One morning it happened by chance that three of the nurses from our team were on the shift together. I was the senior nurse on shift, so was about to start a ward round with one of the consultants. Without warning, I knew that my colleague (and best friend) needed me, in Ollie's room, a corridor away. When I entered the darkened room it was clear that Ollie was close to death. His breathing had slowed to one or two breaths a minute and he was becoming cold and clammy. His mum was sat holding his hands, head bowed over him; talking gently to him, telling him that she loved him and that she would be okay. My colleague was sitting with her, holding her. I reached out and laid my hand on my colleague's shoulder to let her know that I was there with her as he died. We all stayed in physical contact for a few moments. My colleague later expressed she felt so supported when I reached out to let her know that I was there and how important that was to her at that moment – that she was being cared for whilst she cared for Ollie's mum. The physical contact we all had was so important to that moment; rather than just saying that we would be there for each other, we *were* there – in touch with each other.

Later on that day, we washed and dressed Ollie in his favourite football kit – another of his requests – and the rest of his family came to say goodbye. Whilst we were washing Ollie, with a few of the close family in the room, the Catholic priest came in. Unfortunately, in contrast to all the very positive communication we had between us, it seems the priest was unaware that Ollie had died. Because we were washing Ollie he assumed he was still alive, so said to the uncles 'Oh, he's still with us'. There was a moment of horror, where my colleague and I (who could not physically indicate to him as we were washing Ollie) tried desperately to indicate to him with our eyes, and the uncles looked to us. To reassure them, we had to say to him 'No Father, sadly not', and he then came and blessed Ollie, laying his hands on him. He was clearly extremely embarrassed, but spent time with Ollie's uncles, reassuring them that he was sure Ollie's soul was at peace, and retained his composure throughout. He did apologise to us later away from the family, but at the moment he uttered those words our hearts were in our mouths!

51
Intimacy and Relationships: The View from a Hospice

Philip Ball

Introduction

Intimacy and relationships are crucial elements in healthcare, whether in times of good health or in illness. Virtually no one lives in complete isolation; once a person has made the decision to enter into a relationship with the local healthcare system, intimacy between the participants is required in order for benefit to occur. Healthcare culture has developed a model of reliance on trained and competent professionals providing care in one form or another. At the earliest stages there may be some limit over the revelations made, investigations required and actions to be taken; this can escalate as the disease process progresses. Nonetheless, the care is expected to include a focus of respect and dignity aimed at the individual who has deteriorating health.

Once a person has been given a diagnosis and prognosis that is life limiting, intimacy with strangers is likely to become a familiar feature of life. In order to receive care, a person has to become intimate with care providers, surrendering themselves to the processes involved. Not only is this a physical intimacy, it involves becoming exposed in mind and spirit too, in that personal relationships that would normally be protected are open to observation. Issues of intimacy arise for all involved in the life and care of the person; relationships with partners, family members, professionals and with the world around them can be affected. A wider view shows healthcare staff facing issues of intimacy; knowing where boundaries lie through the power they have in relationships with those in their care is one example.

It is the intention here to encourage thinking about intimacy at the end of life, although limited space precludes detailed discussion of all issues. For clarity, the reference to 'care provider' covers any health or social care paid worker, volunteer or family member who provides care to another.

Perspectives on daily living

At our hospice there is an expectation that people under our care will share details of their life with us in the guise of enabling us to provide so-called holistic care. So a relationship develops between each person and the staff at the hospice. As the end of life nears, however, what types of intimacy are of concern to the person in our care, as well to those providing care? What kinds of relationships exist in the last days and hours of life?

For the person who is dying there may be issues to do with physical aspects of life; having help to maintain one's physical body to be clean and comfortable; the insertion of a urinary catheter or having injections lead to situations where nurses, for example, have to have close physical contact with the person in their care. Intimacy becomes woven into the relationship; where there is reluctance or inhibition on the part of the dying person, the nurse may have to use negotiating skills to encourage consideration of further changes to boundaries of acceptable intimacy for that person. Read Joanna's* story below.

Joanna's story: providing intimate care

Many medicines used in palliative care have side effects that can be unpleasant and even dangerous if left unaddressed. One side effect commonly associated with painkillers (analgesics) is constipation. The usual movement of the large intestines is slowed down by these medicines; in addition, a person who is unwell is likely to have a depressed appetite, reduced fluid intake and be less physically active, all of which can make constipation worse. Good practice in palliative care is to use medicines that ease constipation alongside the painkillers. However, towards the end of life these can be less easy to take; a person can therefore develop constipation in a short space of time.

Joanna arrived at the Hospice saying she had abdominal pain, some swelling of her 'tummy' accompanied by nausea. Assessment by the clinicians revealed she had not been able to have a bowel action for some seven days. Examination of her abdomen revealed she was constipated, and after this length of time action was needed. Joanna refused permission for any clinical person to examine her rectum – a process that involves the insertion of a gloved finger via the anus into the rectal area to see if any faeces are present; at the same time the clinician will administer suppositories to try to stimulate the bowel to work if this is judged a necessary intervention.

The hospice clinical team had to begin to negotiate with Joanna; the first step was elucidating her reasons for this refusal, then to ensure that she understood the implications of her decision. Joanna agreed to take by mouth medicines to help stimulate the bowel and soften the stools. This situation was not ideal, as continued constipation can lead to damage to the efficiency of the bowel – blockage by obstructing the bowel. This becomes potentially life threatening unless addressed.

For Joanna the issue was around other people having intimate access to parts of her body in a way that she regarded with some fear and distaste. The nursing team spent the next few days engaged in negotiating with Joanna about this, demonstrating with words and actions, gentleness and sensitivity, when helping Joanna with tasks such as washing and dressing.

Three days after admission, Joanna acknowledged that her condition was not improving as fast as she hoped as she had not managed to have a spontaneous bowel movement. The nurses were able to explain that using suppositories would be a help to stimulate the bowel, giving Joanna time to think over the offer. Joanna agreed the following day to have suppositories. Taking time to explain each step, the nurses were able to insert these and provide to Joanna further evidence that such intimacy might be unusual but can be contained within a relationship of trust between all involved.

A few days later Joanna acknowledged the improvement in her condition brought about by the reduction of the constipation. She also thanked the nurses for the way in which they managed the situation.

---

*All of the names used in this article are pseudonyms.

Physical intimacy with family and friends can also be inhibited at the end of life when the environment either offers no privacy or is not set up to facilitate intimacy. For example, a family member may wish to be near a loved one who is dying and may want to lie next to them; this is something that the hospice will facilitate if that is what is wanted. The urge to be near a dying spouse, for example, can be very strong. To illustrate this, Rhine (2007) tells the story of Jim and Carol. Jim became suddenly very ill while visiting Carol, his wife of 60+ years, as she lay dying in hospital. With his family around him, Jim – having refused potentially life-saving surgery – was able to die holding Carol in his arms following her death only a few minutes before.

A honeymoon has long been associated with the sexual consummation of a marriage. For partners of those who are unwell, a reduced sexual drive can be frustrating even in the short term. The duration of some illnesses can lead to prolonged periods of reduced or no sexual activity. Even kisses and cuddles may be too much to bear because of pain, tiredness, feeling sick and so on. One thing to note is that loss of physical intimacy is something that may give a sense of bereavement and be mourned for some time before the death of the person. Then as the time of death nears, the partner is likely to find themselves in a situation where they can touch, caress and kiss the person. Now read Jack's story.

Jack's story: facilitating physical intimacy

The hospice admitted Jack, who was entering the terminal stage of his lung cancer. Despite saying he wanted to sleep and accepting medication to make him feel drowsy, he remained very restless, often standing up despite the medication he was given. He was most settled when his wife visited and when she held onto him. Jack was a tall man who towered over his wife, so when he was standing up it required a nurse to assist supporting him. This went on for a few hours until Jack no longer had the strength to stand; we were able to him put into bed comfortably where his wife could snuggle up to keep him settled.

However, the facilitation of sexual and physical intimacy within the hospice does also raise moral and ethical dilemmas if the dying person is, or becomes, vulnerable. For example, are intimate acts something that the dying person would consent to if they could? Had there been any physical intimacy before they became unwell? Was such physical contact welcome? In order to protect such vulnerable people, it is important for care providers to discuss this fully to ensure the views of the dying person are respected. Issues of protection arise, and to ensure their own protection some people may choose admission to a hospice for terminal care. In cases of vulnerability, professional teams have to report concerns to those empowered to investigate them. Additionally, the person dying may themselves have been a perpetrator of physical and/or sexual abuse; their death may be viewed with relief by the abused, particularly if they are a family member.

For some people, dying can be a calm affair, slipping away quietly in bed, wheareas others may wish to stand up and approach death with noise and activity. Whatever motivates the dying person in their approach to the final hours and moments of life, they require intimate care set in the framework of a relationship forged in the knowledge that death is not far away for at least one person.

For the dying person there may be a strong desire for other people to hold onto them as they die. This can feel very intimate as life ebbs away; it is human-to-human contact, not a 'professional and patient' interaction. And after death there will be rituals to be gone through for the purpose of preparing the newly deceased person for whatever is expected to happen next. These too are occasions of intimacy, overhung with significance to the spirit and religious beliefs of the deceased person. Death rites or rituals might include washing of the body by specially designated people either because of their gender or religious standing; the application of perfumed oils and burning of incense or similar materials over the body to encourage the cleansing of spirits may be required. Muslims are likely to be dressed in pieces of plain unsewn white cloth that have been worn before whilst on the Hajj. Others may choose to be dressed in the colours of their favourite football team or an outfit that has a special significance. Common rituals involve the use of voice in chanting, prayer or wailing.

In all of this the people providing care have to face the loss of another relationship wherein they had been able to act with intimacy towards their charge. Provision of care involves acts of intimacy: washing a person; feeding them; ensuring that they are comfortable. Bathing appears to hold a particular significance, since in an atmosphere of physical intimacy people will often allow intimate access to their thoughts and feelings and this process can enhance care enormously. Gaining access to family friends and religious leaders involves utilising knowledge gained through intimate conversations. Such conversations must have trust integral to them; the best-practice guidance for conversations involving breaking and discussing 'bad news' include references to conducting such conversations in surroundings that suggest intimacy. These are normally considered to be places that are relatively comfortable; have space to enable people to sit close together or apart, however they might normally do; quiet, where conversations will not be interrupted or overheard; refreshment available if required; with no time pressure. Hospices generally have spaces like this indoors, special rooms or a patient's bedroom. It may be that a conversation takes place in the grounds; taking into account the above criteria, these will still be considered intimate conversations. The place occupied becomes intimate even though it doesn't have any walls or ceilings. It is as though the space becomes intimate rather than just any place. Privacy, confidentiality and respect are names given to the good-practice principles underlying difficult conversations; intimacy is rarely so explicit.

Managing one's own concerns over intimacy and boundaries are important for someone who delivers care. Without sensitivity to others, the care provider will not always engage the critical facility that alerts one to what is appropriate or not in the relationship with the dying person. The care provider can risk leaving unsaid issues of import; for example, the wish to spend time alone with a loved partner, or the desire to create a special message to be delivered before or after death. As they approach death, people will often wish to leave something behind; this may be tokens left in a memory box, letters, or their own DVD that includes, pictures, speech and moving images created by them or with the help of a digital artist. The opportunity to do any of these things may be lost without intimate enquiry by care providers.

Intimacy in care goes together with less physical concerns too. Belief systems may need to be made explicit before death in order for prepare for care after death. These may be challenging to those who provide care; the relationship has to be built based on the ability of both to share the intimacy of beliefs even though there may be no agreement in terms of meaning. A care provider may have a strong belief based on Buddhism, for example, whereas a person in their care could hold a firm conviction in their Christian principles. During discussions about dying and what might happen to a person after death, these two people are likely to hold differing views of the detail; nonetheless, they can agree that something does happen for a person after death.

Care providers may find it difficult to manage their feelings in intimate situations. For example, caring for someone who is seriously disfigured may lead to feelings of revulsion. Clearly, the care provider needs to adopt an alternative response in order to give confidence and comfort to the person concerned. There might also be a strong resonance between the life of the care-giver and that of the dying person, which demands particular control during times of intimacy. Intimate situations are influenced by these, and other, factors; tensions can exist for some people in some situations, whereas not in others. Hospice staff can absorb some of these difficulties through effective team work. In the case of nurses working in the UK, the NMC Code of Conduct (2004) also provides advice on managing such situations.

In practical terms, what does this mean in the hospice? Acts of intimacy go on all the time; it's not just sexual or physically comforting activity, though these are not excluded. Providing a dying person with food and drink can be an intimate act, as can washing them or providing care when they need to pass urine or faeces. Therapeutic massage of hands or feet can soothe someone in distress; finding quiet space for a dying parent to see a child and be able to speak to them are other intimacies. Acts of kindness quietly carried out, or parties provided as a surprise, will often grow out of intimate moments of discussion during the provision of care. Read Peter's story.

Peter's story: the 'Brighton Beach Party'

Peter, a young man in his twenties, wanted to go to the beach with his mates one weekend, but he was no longer well enough to do so. He mentioned it to his care provider one morning, and within a couple of hours his surprise 'Brighton Beach Party' was organised. We had lighthouses, a sand pit, buckets, spades, a wind-break, bunting, a seagull and even a donkey (two staff in costume!), even though we were miles from the sea. Sixty family and friends attended the party and it was a huge success. Three days later, Peter died.

Conclusion

Without intimacy, care for the dying person will be devoid of meaningful acts; indeed, it may not be called care at all. Any resulting relationship would be an impersonal response to needs, instead of an individualised series of intimate moments conducted within a relationship that includes respect for one another and is aimed at respecting the person who has opened up their life to aid those who provide their care.

References

Nursing & Midwifery Council [NMC] (2004) *The NMC Code of Professional Conduct: Standards for Conduct, Performance and Ethics*. NMC, London.

Rhine, David J. (2007) 'The obituary', *CJEM: Journal of the Canadian Association of Emergency Physicians*, 9(2) 136–7.

52
Death in the Early Evening

Tom Heller

Rachel called for a home visit just as evening surgery was about to start. She reported feeling breathless and I knew to go without delay to her house. When I got there her mother was already with her. Rachel was indeed breathless; she asked to get onto the commode. We helped her on and off, after which she lay on her bed in the front room, looked around for a short while, smiled at me and then her mother, stopped breathing, closed her eyes and died. 'Passed away' has become a horrible clichéd phrase but I guess this is what she did.

This event took place more than 25 years ago, and the memory remains quite clear for me. I haven't been present at many people's death since that time, and Rachel, and the way she died, stays with me. Perhaps this episode demonstrated to me the way that I want to die myself; sort of in control and getting the timing and the final farewells just about right.

Rachel was very different from me and certainly came from a sharply contrasting background. A superficial glance at her values and lifestyle might lead you to think that there could never be the basis for a friendship with her doctor. She was a beautician working in the perfume-heavy atmosphere at the entrance to one of Sheffield's department stores. I hate these places. Obviously I am not the target consumer for the sellers of the lipsticks, creams and eye makeup on display. The powerful smell and sanitised displays of expensive, over-packaged stuff feels like an assault to the senses with no redeeming features for me. Most particularly I dislike the painted women also on display. Everyone is forced to walk through their territory to get to other departments. Layered, caked-on makeup and persistent perpetual smiles form a mask behind which who knows what trivial thoughts are running? They certainly know that I won't be stopping at any of their counters and they continue their tittle-tattle with each other as I pass with head down, eyes averted, trying not to breathe in or become contaminated.

But Rachel was one of these people from one of those cosmetics counters and behind the working mask was someone who had quite ordinary thoughts and motives. Most of all she wanted to live and be happy. I don't think she was ever especially philosophical or deep-thinking, and the news of her incurable cancer and inevitable early death came as a horrible shock to her. I think she was a bit younger than I was at the time I became her doctor, but I identified with her shock and shared some of the injustice of it all. Perhaps she could sense that I was identifying with her, and possibly she could see behind my own professional mask? Maybe this wasn't such a difficult task? Doctors think that they have pretty good defences, when in reality perhaps we aren't all that different from mortal humans after all? How would I behave if I ever were to get the privileged chance to know that I am soon going to die? How would I organise my last aliquots of time? Who would I want to be with? What would I want to say to people that I hadn't already said? What lasting memorial would I want to mark my time on earth? Would I be curious about what people thought of me once I was gone?

Since becoming Rachel's doctor, these were the things we talked about for her. Ordinary, mortal concerns. Of course we sorted out issues of pain control and symptom relief, because I don't think that anyone dies from her sort of cancer without the need of some technical medical intervention. But the ordinary, perhaps universal things were far more important, became the currency of our interactions and formed a bond between us. Maybe she knew that I was also rehearsing these questions and answers for myself as we talked about her needs in the months prior to her death? Transference and counter transference, action and reaction, weft and weave. At the back of the tapestry there may be quite a tangle of threads. Was there also sexual attraction? Certainly Rachel asked me to be there at the time of her death and not her husband. He was a professional sportsman away from home at the time trying to establish himself in his chosen sport. There were enough clues that their relationship was not especially close or intimate. She didn't really want him around as she died because she intuitively knew that she would have to look after him and his needs rather than be looked after herself. Goodness, this is heavy stuff for a simple general practitioner to get involved in, but it was her certain choice. He was playing away literally, and she didn't want to upset him or interrupt the progress of his career. Or was I, the doctor, in danger of becoming the idealised husband she never had? Caring, attentive and absorbent of the emotions that spill over and are so important to communicate during terminal illness?

And did I fancy her and take more care of her because of some physical attraction? Would I have made the same efforts for someone I didn't like? Could I have listened so attentively if there was no spark there? It's hard for me to say honestly without getting defensive. Does some form of attraction play a part in the way that any human being looks after another, health worker or not? Sexual or not? Are doctors and nurses in a continual state of denial over this? Is this the elephant in every professional's room? Perhaps we should leave these questions to psychoanalysts with time on their hands to ponder. In any event, Rachel and I liked each other. I looked forward to our consultations and I enjoyed feeling that I was being useful in the face of a tragic situation. Here was a young woman dying and I was sort of enjoying it! Is this how doctors, male doctors at least, get their rocks off, through the misfortune of others?

And what training had I received that might have equipped me for talking to Rachel and having the audacity to think that I could help her? Well, I can't remember the subject of death ever being mentioned at medical school, let alone any discussion of the feelings that might accompany death and dying. I think my influences and any skill came mainly from shared discussions with my peers, from watching district nurses at work and also from non-medical literature. I do remember particularly around this time reading the book *A Way to Die: Living to the End* by Rosemary and Victor Zorza (1980). This wonderful book tells the story of the way that their daughter Jane died aged 25 from malignant melanoma. She did indeed seem to live until the end, but the message of the book is that she needed help and support to do this from her wonderful parents and also from the hospice where she spent her last days. More recently I have learnt from an essay by Judy Gilley (2000), who discusses the intimacy that can be involved during terminal care and the way that people die with the level of intimacy with which they lived. Perhaps the way Rachel died and her exclusion of her husband from this final intimacy tells us something of the way they acted within their relationship?

As death came nearer and Rachel's physical world became smaller, her conscious attention was focussed on her immediate surroundings. Paradoxically wider and deeper concerns became increasingly important to her. I learnt from her that it really is important to find someone with whom to communicate about issues of mortality before it is too late. But none of this is in the medical textbooks, or in the protocols that have sprung up to instruct health professionals about what to do for people as death approaches. We may get paid for keeping a palliative care register and get recognised in other ways for making sure that people are not in pain, but what are the rewards for helping the spiritual journey, of listening to peoples' stories and reflecting with them on the overwhelming beauty of the human condition and their concern for people they are leaving behind?

When I got back to my surgery the reception workers were getting ready to lock up. The evening surgery session was over, but inside several people sat stoically in the waiting area to see me. Determined to get their needs met. Despite being told discretely by the reception workers why my absence from the evening surgery had been necessary, some people waited for my return. I treated their minor viral illnesses, warts and arthritic pains in my usual way with my own mask firmly back in place.

References

Gilley, J. (2000) 'Intimacy and terminal care', in *Death, Dying and Bereavement*. Dickenson, D., Johnson, M. and Katz, J. (eds). London: Sage.

Zorza, R. and Zorza, V. (1980) *A Way to Die: Living to the End*. London: André Deutsch. This is available free at www.zorza.net/resources/waytodie/waytodieTOC.html

Part V
When Someone Dies

Introduction

Sarah Earle and Carol Komaromy

Part V focuses on the feelings and experiences of those who are bereaved. Most of the pieces presented here have been written specifically for this volume and many of the contributors have found it difficult to write about a subject that evokes strong memories and emotions; indeed, some authors have remarked on this within their writing. However, as is to be expected, the feelings and experiences represented here are varied and diverse.

This Part begins with four contributions which explore the immediate and longer term impact of death and bereavement on people's everyday lives. Jacqueline H. Watts writes about the loss of her mother and father at the ages of eight and 23, respectively. Linda Camborne-Paynter reflects on the death of her father when she was only 15 years old, and the subsequent deaths of her brother and mother. In an edited extract from the book *A Grief Observed,* C. S. Lewis writes about his feelings following the death of his wife from cancer; this account has become part of the landscape of grief in modern literature and his book has been presented as a stage play and made into a film. In the last of these four pieces, Keir Hardie writes about the time he attempted to take his own life and his feelings about everyday life since then.

Sudden and unexpected death can create a different form of grief response for some people, and this is explored in the next two pieces. In the first of these, Kythé Beaumont describes the impact on her of her friend's suicide, and in the second piece, Ingrid Nix explores her feelings of grief and bereavement following the death of her beloved dogs, Greta and Mango. Unexpected and sudden deaths are explored further in Part VI of this book.

Many emotions can find expression when someone dies. However, there are powerful expectations that the dominant and acceptable response to death is sadness. The next two pieces challenge this normative expectation and focus on the role of humour within grief and bereavement. First, Ricardo Estee-Wale offers a wry account of his family, the death of his mother, and her funeral and wake in West Africa. Then, Ann Martin reflects on the death of her son Thomas at the age of four and a half. She writes about the importance of humour, the books and friends that offered to 'help', and the source of her great comfort: the 'Hit List' – a list of people that she decided she would never speak to again!

The next selection of pieces explore the importance of communication and, in particular, focus on the role of professional care-givers. First, Gayle Letherby tells the story of her miscarriage (also see Thornton and Letherby in Part VII) and highlights the permanence of the detail of memories at a time of such vulnerability. This account and the one that follows by Josie Hughes, about her grandmother's death and subsequent post-mortem, both highlight the important role of professional care-givers and the potentially damaging effects of poor communication. They Joyce Cavaye takes the professional perspective and uses her first experience of death as a student nurse to consider the extent to which it is possible to prepare professionals to deal with death and dying (also see Heller, Part IV).

The final three pieces of writing in Part V explore the relationship between the private and the public. Firstly, Arnar Árnason writes about the private and public meanings of mortuary rites in Iceland and the proliferation of roadside memorials (also see images in Part I and Dobson in Part VII.) In the next piece, Maxine Birch reflects on the death of her partner and the complexity of contemporary family relationships (also see Hughes in this Part). She writes about her love of flowers and the role of floral tributes as a public recognition of her personal loss. Finally, in the piece by Stuart Todd, attention turns to what Todd describes as 'deaths which are private but not always recognised'. Drawing on a study concerned with the deaths of people with learning disabilities, this piece of writing reports on some of the data from interviews with support workers, bereaved parents and people with learning disabilities. This final piece holds a significant place in this collection, since the grief of people with learning disabilities is so often concealed or denied.

53
Being Orphaned in Early Adulthood

Jacqueline H. Watts

My father, Reginald Jack Bentham (known as Jack), was one of three siblings born into a family who were the coal merchants at Camden Town. In his early forties he met and married a Polish refugee named Halina, settling in Golders Green in north London. My mother was a survivor of the holocaust, having been in Treblinka concentration camp. When my twin sister and I were eight, my mother went to bed one night and died. She was 39 and the victim of a heart attack as well as of the horrors that life had meted out to her. Daddy was devastated, completely and utterly. He never fully recovered from this blow, and neither from the early deaths of his two sisters and best friend that followed soon after.

Somehow we created a re-patterned family unit with love and co-dependence essential to its functioning. We were not well off as daddy had a low-paid job as a clerk in a jute company in the city, but we had enough. We did most things together: opera, cricket and swimming with daddy helping us with our paper rounds at weekends. My sister and I thrived as the years went on, with us both going to university and securing good jobs. In my early twenties I moved to Buckinghamshire because of my work, leaving Mary happily still at home with daddy. Then the call came; daddy had collapsed at London Bridge station on the way to the office and was pronounced dead on arrival at Guy's Hospital. He had had a massive heart attack. He was 63 and my sister and I, 23. Nothing before or since has so profoundly affected either myself or my sister, and now, 30 years on, the sense of irreconcilable loss caused by his early and unexpected death remains.

On being told of his death, we were both numbed by shock and disbelief. There had been no warning, no sign, nothing, and no chance to say goodbye or thank you. I had only seen him a few days before and remember him standing at the gate of our Golders Green family home, a picture of health, tanned and smiling, waving to me as I went off to the last night of the Proms, assuring me he would watch every minute on the telly to see if he could spot me. If I could preserve and keep pristine only one precious memory from my life, it would be the one of me looking back at daddy as I hurried up the hill. And then, a few days later, he was dead. It was beyond belief. At the hospital we sat with him in a side room holding his cold hand, overwhelmed with anguish and grief, hardly able to function at all. Seeing and touching his still, lifeless body was both comforting and traumatic; his physical presence gave us something to hold on to, but his face, without the usual smile, confirmed our new terrible reality. Sitting almost rigid staring at daddy, I can recall an acute physical pain with a tightening across the chest that affected my breathing and an aching sinking hollow feeling in my stomach. When eventually, after some hours, we emerged from the hospital, I will never forget my complete surprise and bewilderment at seeing the buses running and the world outside continuing as usual on a bright sunny early autumn afternoon. But my life would never be the same again.

When daddy was moved to our local undertakers, my sister and I visited him each day and, on the night before the funeral, she spent the whole night with him to, as she said, 'make sure he's not afraid of anything'. The funeral was unimaginably dreadful and the culmination of days of relentless sorrow. The scene of despair abandoned contemporary Western conventions of discrete or elegant mourning, with my sister prostrate on the floor of the crematorium screaming and inconsolable, unable to bear the removal of daddy's body from our midst. I can remember in the evening after the funeral sitting thinking 'This is it now – the rest of my life with no parents', and the prospect of this 'foreverness' sent me into waves of tears and a deep gloom about the future.

At this time and during the months that followed, my grief fluctuated in intensity and took different forms; I was unable to concentrate at work, and the ambitious pathway I had set for myself was abandoned. I withdrew from most social and leisure activities, losing my former love of life and fun. I also lost interest in food, hardly bothering to shop for groceries. So much of both the routine and urgency of life as a young adult became empty and pointless, and my diary entries remind me of my life that was being lived without motivation, especially during the early months of bereavement. I think I was in a kind of 'limbo', with little direction and no plans. Some of my relationships were casualties to this grief that seemed to slightly 'unhinge' me, and I was only able to connect with the intimate group of friends that I had had since infancy (our mothers had together wheeled us as babies to the local clinic, we all started school together and remain firmly together now, 53 years later). Looking back I now know that that was what saved me and continues to save me – their love and, most importantly, the continuity they represent, having always been there from the beginning.

The 'limbo' I have talked about was caused essentially by the loss of 'daughterhood', and instilled within me a sense of panic. This was something I couldn't get used to and it hit me every day adding to feelings of having been 'unrooted', with my inherited history lost to me forever. Expectations for the future that included enjoying time with daddy in his retirement (he only had two years to go before what, for him, was going to be an opportunity for leisure and no work, which he disliked), travelling, watching cricket and just generally being with him were shattered and, for a long time, I couldn't seem to replace these with anything else. I had entered a place called 'disorientation', where there was little meaning to anything that spoke to me of the future. The suggestion, made by a well-meaning colleague a year or so after daddy's death, that I should be beginning to 'get over it' seemed ridiculous because it had not occurred to me that I ever would. In fact, I can still picture the conversation and remember laughing at this comment because it seemed so preposterous. I had settled into a pattern of living with this grief that was always there, not in a morbid way but it was the colour that shaded everything. It felt like a long-held companion, reliable and constant and something I just accepted. It had come almost to feel comfortable.

For years I regularly tried to capture the essence of his presence through 'tuning into' his voice and remembering his 'smell' (he liked 'Old Spice' aftershave!). My sister found particular comfort from taking custody of daddy's ashes, and it was only many years later that we were able to dispose of these over the wicket at the lunch break during a test match between England and Australia (or 'the old enemy', as daddy would say) at his beloved Lord's Cricket ground in London, the place he loved most in all the world. When I watched the fast bowler come in thundering down the wicket over daddy I can recall a sort of joy that, at last, he was where he should be. I don't think this acted as a form of 'closure', but at the time it felt like the completion of another leg of our bereavement journey. And that, really, is what it has been like, all these years – small steps that take me forward in coming to terms with my life that has been characterised and shaped by a series of losses. My grief at his demise is still palpable (this piece has been written in the language of tears) but less intense and much less emotionally disruptive with me now able to reflect positively on his quick death, free of the indignities that so many older people experience in their dying. I suppose, in a way, I have come to a point where I can claim that losing daddy when I did has made me value life, in all its richness, with the imperative to live now and live well, not assuming the certainty of tomorrow.

54
Memories of Death

Linda Camborne-Paynter

I have three memories of death. The first was the summer of 1967. I was 15 years old and my brother was 12. We had just broken up for the summer holidays and over the weekend my parents took us to the local Working Men's Club for a drink. We had a brilliant weekend. However, on the Monday morning my mother woke me quite abruptly at 7 a.m. and said 'Linda, I think your dad's dead'. I remember thinking only old people die or people who are ill, like my granddads, my nan and a couple of my aunts and uncles (my family had seven deaths, including my dad's, in a period of six months). I fell out of bed and ran into their bedroom and found that my dad had died. I knew he was dead because he was deep mauve in colour (not pink like everyone else), so obviously he had been dead for quite a few hours. I went into my brother's room and told him. As my mum wasn't sure what to do I went next door to my neighbour and told her what happened. I didn't have time to get upset as I had to sort things out as my mum was unable to do it. Our dog stayed in the room with dad and I remember having to put his lead on and take him for a walk when the undertaker arrived as the dog would have bitten someone and also I didn't want to see them take my dad away. I had dreams of seeing my mauve dad for a few nights until I was allowed to see him in the chapel of rest. He looked so peaceful and I kissed him on the forehead. However, it was like kissing a block of ice, but at least he wasn't mauve. The dreams never came back.

My next experience of death was in 1974 when my brother was killed. It was about 9.30 in the morning and I was at my desk at work. The phone rang and I answered it. It was one of my neighbours and she said 'Hi Lyn, it's Sis. Your brother's been killed at work'. I remember screaming and someone came into my office and took the telephone from me. I don't remember much after that except my husband suddenly appeared in my office. Obviously someone must have rung him at work and he had come to take me home. My brother and I had had an argument the day before and weren't speaking to each other and I thought 'I can't say sorry now'. He worked for British Rail and had been killed at work. I went to see my brother in the chapel of rest and wished that I hadn't. He didn't look as peaceful as my dad had done and he had a burn mark on his chin. They explained that as he has fallen onto a live rail at work and had died instantly, there was a look of shock on his face that they couldn't disguise. My husband had to go and identify him because my mum and I were not able to. When my husband told me what he had seen (the fact that the burn mark went from his chin right down his body) I was glad that I hadn't gone.

My third experience was when my mum died in 1995. She lived across the road from me and I had a key to her flat. I would check on her every morning and evening to see that she was OK. This particular morning I found mum on the floor. I rang an ambulance and mum was taken to hospital. She had an operation and was soon recovering. She was transferred to another ward as she had tummy problems. She was put in a corner of the ward and one lunchtime when I visited her she had been sick and needed to be cleaned up. I asked one of the nurses and she said that there was no one to do it. I asked for a bowl and did it myself. I put a clean nightie on my mother and then went back to work. Over the next few days my mother's condition got worse and I mentioned this to the nurse on duty. When I visited her at lunchtime she didn't look very well at all. That evening when my husband and I went to see her, my mother had been moved to one of the beds opposite the nursing station, and when I saw my mum I knew that something wasn't right. She had such a far-away glassy look in her eyes, and I didn't want to leave her. As we left I asked if they had my home phone number and when they checked they hadn't, so my husband gave it to them. About 10 p.m. that night we had a call from the hospital. We picked up our daughter and son from their homes and went to the hospital. By the time we got there mum had died. We were led into a room and the doctor explained what had happened. He said that they had been short-staffed – and the locum who had been called in to see my mother didn't know her case – that my mother's condition had deteriorated quicker than they had realised and they were then unable to do anything. I know that my mother didn't have long to live, but to think that the quality of her life at the end was equal to nothing really upsets me. Afterwards we were taken to a side room where mum had been put. Unfortunately they had propped mum up with a pillow and her false teeth had slipped down – she looked like bugs bunny. I didn't want my children to see her because she didn't look very nice, but they wanted to. My daughter was quite upset. A few days later when my mum was in the chapel of rest, I suggested that the family go and see her. She looked so peaceful, and I persuaded my daughter to go and see her. I also took my mum's twin sister to the chapel, and that was a weird experience, looking down at my mum with her twin beside me. It certainly made the undertaker look twice.

Recalling these episodes in my life has been very emotional. I didn't realise until I started to write the details down how much it still upsets me – I have actually been in tears whilst writing this. When my dad and brother died there was nothing I could have done to change the way things had happened, but when my mother died in hospital I felt that I had let her down. The way that she was treated, her quality of life at the end – I wouldn't have treated an animal that way. I did make a formal complaint to the hospital and received a reply which actually asked me to write a letter to the Hospital Trust complaining about the 'lack of resources'. I was livid. Needless to say, I didn't write the letter because I was so angry that my mother had been used as a pawn in a game instead of being treated as a human being who needed care.

55
A Grief Observed

C. S. Lewis

No one ever told me that grief felt so like fear. I am not afraid, but the sensation is like being afraid. The same fluttering in the stomach, the same restlessness, the yawning. I keep on swallowing.

At other times it feels like being mildly drunk, or concussed. There is a sort of invisible blanket between the world and me. I find it hard to take in what anyone says. Or perhaps, hard to want to take it in. It is so uninteresting. Yet I want the others to be about me. I dread the moments when the house is empty. If only they would talk to one another and not to me.

There are moments, most unexpectedly, when something inside me tries to assure me that I don't really mind so much, not so very much, after all. Love is not the whole of a man's life. I was happy before I ever met H. I've plenty of what are called 'resources'. People get over these things. Come, I shan't do so badly. One is ashamed to listen to this voice but it seems for a little to be making out a good case. Then comes a sudden jab of red-hot memory and all this 'commonsense' vanishes like an ant in the mouth of a furnace.

On the rebound one passes into tears and pathos. Maudlin tears. I almost prefer the moments of agony. These are at least clean and honest. But the bath of self-pity, the wallow, the loathsome sticky-sweet pleasure of indulging it – that disgusts me. And even while I'm doing it I know it leads me to misrepresent H. herself. Give that mood its head and in a few minutes I shall have substituted for the real woman a mere doll to be blubbered over. Thank God the memory of her is still too strong (will it always be too strong?) to let me get away with it.

[...]

And no one ever told me about the laziness of grief. Except at my job – where the machine seems to run on much as usual – I loathe the slightest effort. Not only writing but even reading a letter is too much. Even shaving. What does it matter now whether my cheek is rough or smooth? They say an unhappy man wants distractions – something to take him out of himself. Only as a dog-tired man wants an extra blanket on a cold night; he'd rather lie there shivering than get up and find one. It's easy to see why the lonely become untidy; finally, dirty and disgusting.

[...]

I cannot talk to the children about her. The moment I try, there appears on their faces neither grief, nor love, nor fear, nor pity, but the most fatal of all non-conductors, embarrassment. They look as if I were committing an indecency. They are longing for me to stop. I felt just the same after my own mother's death when my father mentioned her. I can't blame them. It's the way boys are.

I sometimes think that shame, mere awkward, senseless shame, does as much towards preventing good acts and straightforward happiness as any of our vices can do. And not only in boyhood.

Or are the boys right? What would H. herself think of this terrible little notebook to which I come back and back? Are these jottings morbid? I once read the sentence 'I lay awake all night with toothache, thinking about toothache and about lying awake.' That's true to life. Part of every misery is, so to speak, the misery's shadow or reflection: the fact that you don't merely suffer but have to keep on thinking about the fact that you suffer. I not only live each endless day in grief, but live each day thinking about living each day in grief. Do these notes merely aggravate that side of it? Merely confirm the monotonous, tread-mill march of the mind round one subject? But what am I to do? I must have some drug, and reading isn't a strong enough drug now. By writing it all down (all? – no: one thought in a hundred) I believe I get a little outside it. That's how I'd defend it to H. But ten to one she'd see a hole in the defence.

It isn't only the boys either. An odd by-product of my loss is that I'm aware of being an embarrassment to everyone I meet. At work, at the club, in the street, I see people, as they approach me, trying to make up their minds whether they'll 'say something about it' or not. I hate it if they do, and if they don't. Some funk it altogether. R. has been avoiding me for a week. I like best the well brought-up young men, almost boys, who walk up to me as if I were a dentist, turn very red, get it over, and then edge away to the bar as quickly as they decently can. Perhaps the bereaved ought to be isolated in special settlements like lepers.

To some I'm worse than an embarrassment. I am a death's head. Whenever I meet a happily married pair I can feel them both thinking. 'One or other of us must some day be as he is now.'

At first I was very afraid of going to places where H. and I had been happy – our favourite pub, our favourite wood. But I decided to do it at once – like sending a pilot up again as soon as possible after he's had a crash. Unexpectedly, it makes no difference. Her absence is no more emphatic in those places than anywhere else. It's not local at all. I suppose that if one were forbidden all salt one wouldn't notice it much more in any one food than in another. Eating in general would be different, every day, at every meal. It is like that. The act of living is different all through. Her absence is like the sky, spread over everything.

[...]

Cancer, and cancer, and cancer. My mother, my father, my wife. I wonder who is next in the queue.

Yet H. herself, dying of it, and well knowing the fact, said that she had lost a great deal of her old horror at it. When the reality came, the name and the idea were in some degree disarmed. And up to a point I very nearly understood. This is important. One never meets just Cancer, or War, or Unhappiness (or Happiness). One only meets each hour or moment that comes. All manner of ups and downs. Many bad spots in our best times, many good ones in our worst. One never gets the total impact of what we call 'the thing itself'. But we call it wrongly. The thing itself is simply all these ups and downs: the rest is a name or an idea.

It is incredible how much happiness, even how much gaiety, we sometimes had together after all hope was gone. How long, how tranquilly, how nourishingly, we talked together that last night!

And yet, not quite together. There's limit to the 'one flesh'. You can't really share someone else's weakness, or fear or pain. What you feel may be bad. It might conceivably be as bad as what the other felt, though I should distrust anyone who claimed that it was. But it would still be quite different. When I speak of fear, I mean the merely animal fear, the recoil of the organism from its destruction; the smothery feeling; the sense of being a rat in a trap. It can't be transferred. The mind can sympathize; the body, less. In one way the bodies of lovers can do it least. All their love passages have trained them to have, not identical, but complementary, correlative, even opposite, feelings about one another.

We both knew this. I had my miseries, not hers; she had hers, not mine. The end of hers would be the coming-of-age of mine. We were setting out on different roads. This cold truth, this terrible traffic-regulation ('You, Madam, to the right – you, Sir, to the left') is just the beginning of the separation which is death itself.

And this separation, I suppose, waits for all. I have been thinking of H. and myself as peculiarly unfortunate in being torn apart. But presumably all lovers are. She once said to me, 'Even if we both died at exactly the same moment, as we lie here side by side, it would be just as much a separation as the one you're so afraid of.' Of course she didn't *know*, any more than I do. But she was near death; near enough to make a good shot. She used to quote 'Alone into the Alone.' She said it felt like that. And how immensely improbable that it should be otherwise! Time and space and body were the very things that brought us together; the telephone wires by which we communicated. Cut one off, or cut both off simultaneously. Either way, mustn't the conversation stop?

Unless you assume that some other means of communication – utterly different, yet doing the same work, would be immediately substituted. But then, what conceivable point could there be in severing the old ones? Is God a clown who whips away your bowl of soup one moment in order, next moment, to replace it with another bowl of the same soup? Even nature isn't such a clown as that. She never plays exactly the same tune twice.

It is hard to have patience with people who say 'There is no death' or 'Death doesn't matter'. There is death. And whatever is matters. And whatever happens has consequences, and it and they are irrevocable and irreversible. You might as well say that birth doesn't matter. I look up at the night sky. Is anything more certain than that in all those vast times and spaces, if I were allowed to search them, I should nowhere find her face, her voice, her touch? She died. She is dead. Is the word so difficult to learn?

I have no photograph of her that's any good. I cannot even see her face distinctly in my imagination. Yet the odd face of some stranger seen in a crowd this morning may come before me in vivid perfection the moment I close my eyes tonight. No doubt, the explanation is simple enough. We have seen the faces of those we know best so variously, from so many angles, in so many lights, with so many expressions – waking, sleeping, laughing, crying, eating, talking, thinking – that all the impressions crowd into our memory together and cancel out into a mere blur. But her voice is still vivid. The remembered voice – that can turn me at any moment to a whimpering child.

56
Suicide

Keir Hardie

In some ways I find it hard to imagine why anyone would want to kill themselves, and yet I once tried to, less than ten years ago, but my perspective was very different at that time. These days I think that life is so short that even if it's terrible it's over soon enough, but that's not how things seem to the deeply miserable. When mental pain is so intense that you can't see anything else you only see things as part of the pain, you can't see outside it, if you could you'd be able to put things into perspective better.

Even as I tell you this I can't tell you how bad it was, it is beyond my imagination. I can remember doing it, but I can't think of why really. Nothing that adds up. I'm glad to have forgotten but surprised at how well I have, and I can't be sure whether my 'insights' about what was going on for me at the time are really that or just theories that I've become sold on. But it was much nearer the time when I first started talking to people about these ideas, so that gives me some confidence. Also some of the things I think about my experience seem so compelling to me as true about those who attempt or complete suicide that I often say that it's like this or that for 'us', and they're not things I've backed up with a survey, just my perspective, the perspective of someone who's been there as seen from a long way away.

It's impossible to say where it all started, nobody ever can. There are countless events, thoughts and feelings that lead someone to that point, and if some of them had happened differently … but anyway, I was very miserable for many years, so there I was, in this big hole. I can't recall the specifics of the pressures on me at the time: poverty, loneliness, depression, homelessness. I once tried being more specific to oblige a journalist, and after a few minutes I realised that I had been getting mixed up with some other miserable time, but these are all things that at various times led to me feeling trapped, out of options. Feeling out of options is a very dangerous thing for someone who feels that their life is irredeemably unbearable. I don't personally now believe that anyone wants to die as such, not in itself, but that for some people sometimes it can seem like the closest thing they can come up with to a solution to what they are facing. Many people have these thoughts from time to time, but only a few of us go further and get the intention to do it for any length of time. I was no exception, I don't know what was different that time, I think it may have been at least partly down to dangerous thoughts. I remember that once I decided to do it I felt stupid for not having done it much sooner, I wouldn't have had to go through a lot of stuff.

My next moves weren't very typical from what I can gather, there was a chilling logic to it all, the logic of a distorted world, things that were all logical given the assumptions but there was no internal critic to say 'no, but …'. I didn't hide my intentions from services because I knew they couldn't section me or anything just for being suicidal, I knew I'd have to be ill too, and I didn't seem ill at the time. It's common for people in that situation to seem much improved, having made the decision and being finally spared from all the distressing 'will I, won't I?' internal debates. Having entertained thoughts of wanting to be dead all those times and then done nothing, I was concerned for my resolve, but I was quite happy to let the psychiatrists check me out because I didn't want to do it if I was only wanting to do it because I was nuts, that would be foolish, if it was that, then they could deal with it.

Unfortunately they felt that I was suicidal but not ill, so there was nothing they could do, but they'd rather I didn't. This strengthened my resolve and helped to back me into a corner, which I needed to do, it was one less option. It wasn't their fault, they were just doing their jobs within the limitations of those jobs. They could only go on how I was presenting. Most of the people who say they're going to do it don't, and they have to draw the line somewhere. It's an uncomfortable truth, but there are a lot of people doing a lot of suffering right now, and there's only a very small cross-section of human suffering that the welfare state makes much effort at dealing with. They have to prioritise, however they see fit at the time. And so a lot of people are suffering and feeling trapped right now, in a mess that they could be got out of, which they could get themselves out of, perhaps, if they had the resources, and nothing will be done. It seems pretty awful, but it's hard to imagine that things could ever be any different. It can't have gone in my favour; the great difficulty I was having in choosing a method – I had rejected everything I had thought of, too much of a downside. It's one of the big risk assessment things they use to decide if you're really going to do it or not, planning. The more detailed a plan you have, if you have one at all, the more likely you are to do it. Or the more points you get – they mark on various factors then add up the points to see how you did.

So that was that, where to now? Out of other options, I fell back on a method I'd already rejected and decided on an overdose of painkillers. I had to go to several shops to buy enough now they limit the number you can buy at once. Although it didn't stop me, it's a good idea and it has saved lives, plenty of people having a bad night overdose on whatever they have in the house. I had no idea how many to take, that was one of the reasons I'd already rejected the method. So I took a lot, and I took them over several hours with food, and some of them were soluble ones in water, because I didn't want to bring any up. I deliberately avoided thinking about anything that would weaken my resolve, like those that loved me and the mess I'd leave behind, so I wouldn't have to deal with it. There's a lot about not being able to deal with things in this story. I still find it a bit shocking that I was able to do that, to deliberately put those things out of my mind. And then I went to sleep.

I woke up at around 6 a.m. with terrible stomach cramps; I think I decided pretty quickly to go to A&E, and I was in hospital for six days until they stopped being worried about my liver's gamma count or something. That's something else that still seems pretty shocking to me, six days seems like a pretty bad one. Within a few days I wasn't sure if I wanted to be dead or not anymore. I think that knowing I could do it made a difference to me, I think it motivated me more to take care of myself mentally and avoid being vulnerable to outside forces in any way. After a year or two in supported accommodation for homeless people I got a council flat, and I don't think you can get any more secure than that. That has made a big difference to my ability to create a situation for myself where I'm pretty content. I don't have a fantastic life now, too poor, but it's not bad, and I don't like the idea of dying at all; in fact, I resent the fact that I will eventually. It cramps my style, there are so many things I'd be doing if I wasn't so aware of how limited our time on Earth is, so many books I'd read, paintings I'd paint, but as it is I don't make the time. I seem to have gone from one extreme to the other, when it comes to perspective, but this is by far the nicer end of the telescope.

57
Suicide is Painless?

Kythé Beaumont

I have no idea where I was when Elvis died, even less idea when Kennedy was assassinated. But I remember vividly where I was when the phone rang and I heard that my friend had killed herself.

Looking at those words on the page as I write, it's hard to choose the right words – the phrase 'killed herself' seems so much more violent, more 'in your face', more 'sudden' than 'committed suicide'. I don't know why that is, but her death was sudden and it was unexpected.

When she died (that word sounds even more distant than 'killed herself') I had moved 200 miles away from the city and from the wide group of friends that we were both part of. We had been good friends. We were there for each other. This was an era of optimism and great change. As part of the wider group we felt we could change the world. When I moved I felt distant from the social change that had been going on around us. But we were not distant in terms of friendship. We talked on the phone and she came to visit several times. Sometimes she would be on her own, sometimes with others. She met, liked and socialised with our new friends in our new town. During those times we would talk. Really talk. Deep intense discussions. And yet I had no idea.

When the news came, my partner and I needed to be there back in familiar places and with old friends. We jumped in the car and got to where people who knew her were gathering. There was a lot to do and a lot to discuss. Some friends were on holiday abroad and we needed to contact them. They needed to know and we needed them to be there with us. Being together and sharing was important. It brought people together emotionally, even though physically we weren't a cohesive group. At that time we were shocked – we couldn't believe it, but possibly we could. Being together meant we could grieve together, and those who were about in our friend's last days began to replay what had happened to see if they could find a sign that this was going to happen.

On one level I still couldn't believe it. I needed more information. We tried to imagine those last few days, hours, moments. We needed to make sense of it somehow. We needed to piece it together.

I think probably at an early stage I became resigned to thinking that if my friend was ill and things were out of control, this making a decision to take her own life (another phrase to describe what actually happened) and then acting on it was one way she had of taking control back. She was being very powerful. We were in the height of involvement in the Women's Liberation Movement and taking control of our own bodies and our own lives was important. We had read 'Our Bodies Ourselves' – a feminist handbook for health – examined parts of our own bodies we had never seen before, and shared different ways of caring for our health, so for our friend to take control of her own death felt part of this. This helped me accept what she had done. It all made sense – or did it?

I still needed more. I remember thinking about the phrase 'bearing witness'. I needed to know this had happened. I needed to believe it had happened. I went with a friend to see her at the undertakers. I don't think she was dressed in her own clothes and her body in the coffin was almost smothered by the satin. It was at a time when no self-respecting feminist would be seen dead in make-up. My friend was wearing make-up. She didn't particularly look peaceful, didn't particularly look 'at peace'. She didn't look like my friend. It felt like it wasn't her. It felt as though she wasn't there.

During the time before the funeral I saw her everywhere – in the most unusual places. The car park in my new town – what was she doing there? Why was she pushing a trolley round my local supermarket 200 miles away? Getting closer, it wasn't her, but she was there, I could feel it. I could sense it. I remembered long forgotten conversations we had had in minute detail, things that we had done together years ago as though it was yesterday. Memories that I never thought I had.

The funeral was huge. There were lots of flowers outside the crematorium. I don't remember the service but I remember seeing many people from my past that I had lost touch with. I was in shock and it was good that they were there. But it was also confusing. I was glad to see my friends but so sad to be there.

Later, at home, I thought back to one of the times my friend came to stay with us after I had moved away. She drove with me to a hospital where I visited another friend who had tried to kill herself. On the long way back I talked – she listened. I was very upset. I wanted to do something. I felt powerless to help. Sharing that experience with her at that time was important. I felt she understood how that suicide attempt affected me. I hoped she knew somewhere how her suicide might be affecting me now.

Back then, I wasn't sure if I believed in life after death, or where people go when they die. I am even less sure now I am older. I am not religious and don't have it clearly mapped out in my mind. Sometimes I think that people live on in the memories of others after death. In other, more muddled, times I believe that a person's soul (and I am not sure what that is as a non-religious person) moves on to the body of another. I certainly don't think dead people are sitting about on clouds or chatting casually with Elvis or JFK. But I did hear her speak to me after she was dead. I have never heard a voice like that before or since. I am not even sure why I believe it was her, because of course I don't believe in 'this sort of thing'. I was just about to go to sleep one night, I hadn't been thinking about her and suddenly I heard her voice calling my name, exactly how she spoke. 'I am alright', she said. And I knew she was.

Time has passed and I still think of her – she is still with me in my head, in my memories. How would it be now if she was still alive? I am not sure. Would we still be friends? I would like to think so.

58

The Loss of Mango

Ingrid Nix

I used to have two dogs, Greta (a Giant Schnauzer) and Mango (a Mini Schnauzer). I got both dogs (two-year-olds) from my mother, who bred them. In that sense, they also represented a part of her life (and obsession). My siblings, each in different ways, valued the dogs because of this link which bound the family.

I got Mango two years after Greta, so that they could be company for each other. Greta was my favourite, my wonderful trusty companion, my first experience of unconditional love. She paid me the compliment of noticing when I was absent and welcoming me when I returned. She lived through many of my adventures and trials and was my steadfast solace when things went pear-shaped. When she started to age I didn't molly-coddle her. I always took care of her during bigger illnesses but I think the smaller, day-to-day developments perhaps got absorbed into the bigger events of my own life. Perhaps because she was big, like me, I expected her to tough things out.

When on holiday in France, Greta had an accident, falling in the dark in unfamiliar terrain; it was clear to me within hours that she was not going to recover, due to paralysis. I had a couple of terrible days on my own trying to decide what to do, with one of my sisters on the phone supporting me through it. Eventually I did the terrible deed, and had her put down in the back of my car. I wept and howled on the way back home without her, but somehow in the weeks and months ahead managed, with Mango there, to focus on the new way forward. Suddenly Mango came to the fore, having been obscured by Greta's larger presence.

The next few years I got to know him on his own. Sadly, he developed physical problems and I had to care for him, see him through difficult operations and gradually more and more debilitating conditions. I started to feel I understood what it must be like to look after a human long term. He was dependent on me, I was his principle carer. Every aspect was mediated through me acting on his behalf. As time progressed I was constantly faced with the torment of watching him, wondering if or how he was suffering. Each day or part of a day I had to work out logistics, who would care for him while I was at work, or for example, whether I could leave him while I went out for a meal. In fact I took him everywhere, including to work, weather permitting. I'd be thinking about where I could find shade to park him in and how I could take him for a walk (or hobble) between meetings.

Eventually, I had to face making the decision to have him put down. By this time I was exhausted and raw from the emotional strain. The weekly deadlines I kept setting myself, to see how he managed, now became days. Eventually I set it to be a Friday afternoon. I wanted to have time to recover so I could face work on Monday. How awful to think of something so practical. I arranged to have the vet come to my home. The night before, I had slept with my head at the foot of my bed so I could be closer to Mango's basket. I slept with the blind up so we could lie in the moonlight. That hot summer morning I'd put him out in the garden under the shade of a tree on the patio so he could be in nature. Poor thing wet his bed. I had, for months, had to hold him on his legs to help him go to the toilet. This was the first time he had soiled himself. For me it was a sign that his body was giving up. I freshened his bed. When the vet and her assistant came I put him in the cool of the kitchen. What touched me was that the assistant also wept. When she picked him up afterwards she wrapped him in a towel they had brought and carried him like a child away in her arms. I was so grateful she understood some of my pain so I didn't have to apologise or feel self-conscious.

The days and weeks ahead I walked along our frequented paths. I wanted to remember and relive, in private. I would sit on the bench where we would stop. I was afraid of the process which would come, of losing, forgetting. With time it has become too painful because I can't go there without seeing him struggle on his weak legs, or see him fall without being able to get up. Instead I have photos of him in my bedroom, in a CD case in my car, on the wall of my study. I use his and Greta's names as my computer passwords. When I accidentally drop pasta on the floor, when I chop the ends off carrots, I think of Mango who would been given these in his bowl. Strange thing is, I have barely any photos of my mother on display. I do use her date of birth as one of my PIN numbers and have things from her house, such as crockery and furniture, and some clothes.

I wonder whether my deeper sense of loss for Mango was because I perceived him as more vulnerable and therefore felt a greater sense of responsibility for him. I feel a bit like a parent who has lost a child. The sense of smallness of Mango puts him in a different relationship to me than Greta, who was big. Also because his illness and condition eked it out of him, instead of Greta's accident which almost dictated what should happen, it made the process a drawn-out period of slow pain and approaching loss.

I wrote a poem the afternoon of his death, sitting on our bench, and then a year on to mark the anniversary. This year I didn't – I was overseas on a holiday, something I seldom managed during 15 years of having the dogs. Although I feel bad that I am forgetting to make specific dates for remembering them, I can tell you that writing this has caused a pile of tissues to appear alongside me on the desk.

59
The Death of a Socialite

Ricardo Estee-Wale

Mark Anthony's famous eulogy to Julius Caesar contains the often quoted words: 'Friends, Romans, countrymen, lend me your ears; I come to bury Caesar, not to praise him; The evil that men do lives after them. The good is oft interred with their bones,' (Shakespeare, *Julius Caesar*, III: ii). In West Africa, death is looked at in a different light. If one's family is able to throw a fabulous wake, where there is a feast of Babet's proportion and a fountain's supply of alcohol, then all is forgiven. I found to my surprise that death and the subsequent funeral is more often than not a competition between the living relatives, as to who can throw the biggest party.

I still remember the death of my grandfather in 1979. He was a millionaire and it seemed like the whole town had come to pay their last respects on the day of the funeral. He had 17 children from his five wives and each of them tried to outdo each other in the glamour and wealth stakes – whether they could afford it or not. It was 'mandatory' that all his children each slaughtered a cow or two in his honour. My mother was not to be upstaged. She got the most expensive lace and brocade material for my sisters and I, new shoes and watches (and the cow). She was not going to let any of her siblings' children beat us in the glamour stakes. My uncles and aunts all took out centre-page ads in the obituary columns of the national dailies. One of my uncles made sure that he had BA Honours after his name. My mother made sure that everyone knew that my sisters and I lived in England, which was extra kudos on the one-upmanship stakes. I was quite young at the time so these intricacies and micro-politics passed me by. I just remember eating to excess without really feeling sad for my departed grandfather; to be totally honest, I didn't really know him. Saying that, no one else looked that distraught either. As Bing Crosby was dreaming of a White Christmas, my mother and her siblings were undoubtedly thinking of the potential massive inheritance. This later caused a big squabble between them because the will got 'lost' and so the older siblings divided houses and land out 'equally' between them all. Being one of the youngest, my mother got a flat, which was quite a good slice of the 'fortune' since my grandfather had 37 properties!

It was my mother's turn in 2001. My mother died unexpectedly at the age of 56 in West Africa. She was feeling a lot of pain in one of her legs (it was a blood clot), to the extent that the people around her advised her to seek medical help. Unfortunately, the medication she was given made her feel worse. So, some elders from her church – rather than take her back to the hospital – decided to pray for her. Unfortunately the prayers did not work and so when she suffered a massive heart attack, they panicked, placed her on her bed and fled. I suppose it must have been her time to go because neither medicine nor prayers could have saved her that day.

As the eldest child it was up to me to arrange the funeral. First of all I had to fly over and identify the body. The autopsy had already been done and I thought that her body would have been preserved like the ones seen in hospital dramas – where the corpse just looks like a person sleeping.

Such dramas depict very clean mortuaries where a sympathetic orderly or pathologist pulls the corpses out of a pristine refrigeration unit. What I was to find shocked me greatly. Two burly men, with all the delicacy and sensitivity of a circus prize-fighter, pulled this naked body out of an iron drawer which looked more like the driftwood one collects after a heavy storm. The body was almost unrecognisable. 'This is your mother' I was informed in a very matter-of-fact way. The socialite, the daughter of a millionaire, was a mangled and forgotten carcass stripped of all dignity.

It has made me wonder ever since why we mortals strive to stay young, live longer and look beautiful if there is a very strong likelihood that we will end up looking like driftwood anyway. My mother was always using the most expensive creams, lotions, potions and perfumes, but there was no evidence of that when the body was produced. If we are lucky enough to escape that driftwood fate we will either end up on a burning furnace and barbequed to ashes, kept in an awful urn or have one's ashes scattered on some forsaken football ground. There is, however, the greener option – get buried and become fodder for the worms and fertilizer for the soil. Due to the fact that no real heat is produced, it doesn't add to global warming like the fiery furnace option.

I still remember the glee on the faces of the hangers-on when I arrived. 'This guy is from England he must have lots of money to spend whilst here', they must have thought and expected. I was shown a coffin that cost hundreds of pounds but I opted for the cheapest plywood coffin, to some people's utmost disgust. No matter how much the coffin costs they are all bio-degradable, I reasoned; so why should I spend hundreds of pounds on a coffin that will meet the same fate as the cheapest option? My uncle said that a woman of my mother's social standing should not be shamed in such a way. I assured him that as she was dead my mother knew nothing about it.

The elders of the church who had previously prayed for her (and failed!!) offered to say some special prayers for my mother (for a token 'donation') to the church. I declined. I said 'She's dead, your prayers won't bring her back, in fact your prayers didn't work when she was alive.' I then quoted the Bible, 'And it is appointed unto men once to die, but after this comes judgement (Hebrews, 9:1).' That kept them quiet.

My uncles asked how many cows my sisters and I would be slaughtering in honour of our mother. Our response was that we would go the local butchers and buy enough meat for the wake that was to follow afterwards. They were none too pleased because I had potentially cut them off from half a year's supply of free meat.

It was also expected that live musicians be gathered to sing her praises. I said a hi-fi and CDs would suffice. At this time I was becoming a major obstacle and irritant to all concerned.

Where my sisters and I were 'stung' was in church, where all the charities and clubs my mother was the chair of came for donations. This was fast becoming a battle between 'Ricardo and sisters' verses 'the money grabbers'. The battle in the church was won by the money grabbers, but my sisters and I won the overall war.

The best was still to come. My uncle (my mother's younger brother) confessed to my sister that what hurt him the most about my mother's death was that she had just promised him £13,000 that week. If that wasn't a hint, I wonder what was? My sister replied 'Well, that's life'; I corrected her and said 'no, that's death'; it has a funny way of mucking up one's mortal plans.

My sisters and I left for England the next day. As we were flying over the Pyrenees, two scriptures from the Bible came to my mind: 'Vanity of vanities! All is vanity' (Ecclesiastes, 1: 2) and 'For what is your life? It is even a vapour, that appeareth for a little time, and then vanisheth away' (James, 4:14).

I wonder what my funeral will be like? I have a niggling feeling that all expenses will be spared.

60
Black Humour and the Death of a Child

Ann Martin

'Your son, Thomas, has died. Does he have any clean clothes with him? It is urgent!' These were the words of the French doctor at the hospital in the Dordogne where Thomas, aged four and a half, had been taken following a swimming accident. I already knew he was dead, he had to be, he'd been missing for about half an hour, and we then knew he'd been under the water for most of that time. So the doctor telling us that wasn't really a shock, but why would he need clothes? My mind went into a spin trying to picture possible scenarios in which a dead child would need to be appropriately dressed. I came up with no sensible suggestions to myself. Does it sound weird to be have been momentarily gripped by a surreally funny thought in the midst of one of the most awful experiences life can offer? It probably does, but I discovered that death, possibly more than any other life event, is full of wildly ranging emotions and humour is very much one of them.

In fact, humour was a key emotion I felt quite randomly but very sharply during those early minutes, hours, days, weeks and months following Thomas's death, and I learned to regard it as a few minutes of welcome and necessary respite from the other long periods of terrible pain and numbness. Most of the time, my four-year-old son was dead, nothing could ever be right again, and I couldn't see how I would ever be able to find any aspect of life anything more than bearable at best. And then, a comment or even sometimes a difficult situation, would make me laugh and for a moment I felt a bit better.

Reading the helpful books for bereaved parents (they're mainly not!) did in fact trigger some amusement. I read endlessly about all the different stages of grief which were 'absolutely normal' and then I was able to tell myself I was in the 'angry' phase, or the 'acceptance' phase or the … but so what ? I made myself laugh analysing every emotion as it happened, almost like endlessly re-winding a video or DVD to see the same thing over and over. In the end, I decided it best to just feel what I felt without thinking about it too much!

People were kind, of course, but not all of them! I did experience the classic incident of an acquaintance running down the other supermarket aisle to avoid me, but us both being aware that she had seen me and that I had seen her avoidance tactics too! Was I upset – no, I thought it was quite funny that she had got into such a state about seeing me – I didn't want to see her either. And that was the beginning of the Hit List, which was source of great comfort to me during that first year. My Hit List consisted of names of people I decided that I would NEVER speak to again. I gave myself permission to be quite ruthless – the woman at playgroup, the neighbour over the road, a former colleague, and it really cheered me up to think that now I realised that life could be changed or ended so fundamentally at one short stroke, it was just too precious to be wasted on perfunctory conversations with people you really don't like. Honestly, the people I have never spoken to since! The pleasantries I've avoided!

Frank was someone I did speak to again, because he was a major distraction on a bad day, so I do thank him for that. Frank was quite a kind neighbour, who came round shortly after we got home without Thomas to say how terribly sad he was. He was desperate to tell us that we only had to ask if there was anything, *anything* at all that he could do to help. So we did ask. Frank was very proud of his garden and spent much of his retirement planting, weeding and mowing. Could he mow our small strip of lawn for us prior to the funeral as our mower was broken? The response was stunning – he hadn't meant 'that kind of help'! I think we may well have laughed in front of him, but in any case we did laugh a lot when he'd gone. The mystery was – what sort of help did he mean then? Counselling, a bottle of whisky, knowing that he 'was there for us' (but not in the garden)?

Sharon, too, was funny. Having had four children at the start of my summer holiday and coming home with only three of them was a difficult situation for any friend or visitor to handle. I knew that, of course, and often tried to help people out by moving the conversation on to 'safe' ground. I was often tired, though, and sometimes just not able to do that. Sharon could see I was having a bad day – I could see she wished she hadn't come round, but she had and I was grateful. In an attempt to search for the positive in any situation, however, Sharon proclaimed that only having three children now would, in fact, make it much easier for me in the mornings with less children to get ready. Yes, Sharon, every cloud … ! Was I upset at what she'd said? No. Did I laugh? Yes, a lot, and it did me good, I'm sure.

Thomas died during our summer holiday. People seemed to focus on it a lot – often commenting it was a terrible time for that to have happened. Just occasionally, I would reply: What – ten past six? A Wednesday? Better in the winter do you think? Not to make anyone feel uncomfortable but really just to let them see I could laugh still, even and maybe especially about Thomas who always did make me laugh.

The surreal nature of the events surrounding a bereavement can be quite funny: drawing up a list of things to do included 'collecting the ashes' on one occasion, 'phone Interpol' on another, alongside the usual 'clean floor, buy cat food'. Finding some black marks on the back of my car seat where Thomas had kicked it in a temper a few weeks before and then being annoyed about it was a good day too!

A year later, I had another baby – a girl after four boys. Really, really lovely, but not making things 'right' of course. I have evidence in the form of New Baby cards of so many people's good wishes – nice of course – but suggesting that they were 'so thrilled things have worked out' or 'you've got an even number of children again' (yes handy!) or even 'a baby girl – so glad – make up for everything!' Well, no, actually my son is still dead and I still miss him. Who are these people?

Some years on, humour and bereavement are still closely connected in my mind. I think bereaved parents especially are dangerously 'edgy' in a way. Nothing can be said or done that is ever as bad as what's happened, so it makes it easy to stand aloof from people and situations and be disconnected from the social norms and etiquettes – we can be outrageous or cynical or silent and moody. And we can laugh if we want to, at whatever we find funny. This is a strength, both for us and everyone else, because we can be tearing down the barriers between the bereaved and the non-bereaved and helping people to see us as essentially the same people but having changed lives.

… and Thomas needed clean clothes as a French traditional mark of respect for a dead body!

61
Experiences of Miscarriage

Gayle Letherby

Definitions of miscarriage:

- A spontaneous abortion: a pregnancy that terminates on its own prior to birth.
- Spontaneous delivery of a foetus (developing unborn offspring) before it is able to live on its own.
- Spontaneous loss of a viable embryo or foetus in the womb.
- Failure of a plan …

It's hard to find a definition of miscarriage that gets close to representing how I felt and feel about the *death of my baby*. Only the last in the above list gets anywhere close. As a girl and young woman I fully expected and wanted to become a mother to lots of children. Although, growing up as an only child, I was vaguely aware of the fact that my parents had intended to have more children and that this had 'just never happened', I thought little about the consequences of this for my mother and father. I enjoyed being an only child, and felt loved and cherished by my parents, even though I didn't seem to receive the material or emotional benefits that stereotypes of only childhoods told me I was entitled to.

In 1979 I married: I was young, just 20 years old. The wedding took place just ten days after my qualifying as a nursery nurse and six months after the death of my beloved father (see Thornton and Letherby in Part VII). My subsequent jobs, first as one of three nursery nurses in the postnatal ward of a large London hospital and next as second-in-command in a university day nursery (also in London), felt like preparation for my inevitable role as earth mother. I felt smugly prepared for parenthood, and argued that all parents would benefit from the training and experience that I had gained. In addition I was sure that I was a 'natural', and a couple of years into marriage I was more than ready to start 'trying for a family'. My husband was less keen but I eventually persuaded him and early in 1983, having read an article in a magazine that it was important for us to be healthy before contemplating pregnancy, I booked an appointment at the GP's for us so that we could both have a pre-parental check-up. The doctor seemed amused by our concerns and did little but offer advice on healthy eating and living.

It was 15 months before I became pregnant, and I remember the feelings of desperation and helplessness and the growing sense of grief and loss as month after month the blood in my knickers meant no pregnancy yet. March 1984 though was a joyful month, I was pregnant! A pregnancy test confirmed it and I enjoyed gaining weight, suffering back-ache, being sick and preparing for our new arrival. Between weeks 10 and 15 the sickness stopped and my weight gain slowed too. I was a little anxious but told no-one, convincing myself that everything was fine. A visit to the local hospital for my first scan changed everything, though. It appeared that our baby wasn't growing and was only of nine weeks' gestation, but as I'd lost a little blood at weeks four and eight we were told not to worry too much: 'Maybe your dates are different than you think.' Sent away and told to come back a week later, I retreated to the sofa, terrified of moving, frightened of what might come next. Back to checking my knickers for blood, I didn't have to wait long and a couple of days later I started to bleed and experience cramps in my lower back. In bed that night, sleeping lightly against the pain, I woke needing to go to the toilet. As I stood, what seemed to me and to my husband like gallons of bloodied water gushed from me. Once in the bathroom I felt the urge to push, and when I stood up a tiny foetus, my baby, our child, was in the toilet. I wrapped him or her (we never found out the sex) in a towel and we rang the emergency doctor's number and were told that I had obviously 'lost the baby' (how careless of me!) so the best thing was to get some sleep and call the surgery in the morning. This was followed by several hours of cramps, horrendous pain and passing of large clots of blood. My husband wanted to call the doctor again but I stubbornly and angrily refused: 'They told us to wait until morning, so we will.' Who was I angry with, I wonder? The doctor, certainly; myself as well, and probably every woman who had ever had a baby. I slept at last early in the morning and on waking rang the doctor's surgery to ask to speak to a doctor and for a home visit. The receptionist did not want to put me through at first and I had to detail the experiences of the night before she deemed it serious enough for the doctor's attention. A couple of hours later, a doctor I'd never met before appeared at my bedside. He examined me and proclaimed me well enough not to have to go to hospital. He left then, taking away with him the remains of the baby and some of the clots I'd keep for him to see.

Over the next days I grieved at home, receiving comfort from my husband, my mother, some close friends and my cats. After ten days, as instructed, I went to the same doctor for the check-up he had booked me in for in my bedroom the last time we had met. Expecting a sympathetic welcome, I was distressed and angry when it was obvious that he had forgotten who I was.

Nine months later, after nine more monthly crying episodes in the toilet, I returned to the doctor's office once more. This time I saw a different GP who told me that 'getting upset won't do any good, you just have to relax'. Several months after that at yet another visit, the possibility of 'infertility'* treatment was mentioned for the first time. The doctor spoke of sperm tests and in-vitro fertilization although with reference to the latter wondered out loud if this might be 'going a bit too far'.

Throughout this (largely) negative medical experience, I grieved for the baby I had lost and began to grieve for those I thought I would never have. I resigned from my job – at the time of my miscarriage I was working as a daily nanny to a 6-year-old girl – and undertook various administrative jobs for the next couple of years. Feeling that I might not ever want to return to nursery nursing, in September 1985 I went to my local college of Further Education to improve

---

*I write 'infertility', 'involuntary childlessness' and 'voluntary childlessness' in single quotation marks to highlight problems of definition. For further information and to see some of my work on reproductive identity and non-parenthood, see Letherby, G. (1993) 'The meanings of miscarriage' *Women's Studies International Forum* 16:2; Letherby, G. and Williams, C. (1999) 'Non-motherhood: ambivalent autobiographies' *Feminist Studies* 25:3; Letherby, G. (1999) 'Other than Mother and Mothers as Others: the experience of motherhood and non-motherhood in relation to "infertility" and "involuntary childlessness"' *Women's Studies International Forum* 22:3; Exley, C. and Letherby, G. (2001) 'Managing a Disrupted Lifecourse: issues of identity and emotion work' *Health* 5:1; Letherby, G. (2003) 'I didn't think much of this bedside manner but he was very skilled at his job: medical encounters in relation to "infertility"' in Earle, S. and Letherby, G. *Gender Identity and Reproduction: social perspectives* London: Palgrave; Earle, S. and Letherby, G. (2007) 'Conceiving Time?: Women who do or do not conceive' *Sociology of Health and Illness* 29:2.

my typing skills. I also decided to sign up for a Psychology O-Level, just for interest. But when the psychology option did not run, due to lack of numbers, the tutor persuaded me to sit in on the A-level Sociology session. From the beginning I found Sociology both stimulating and challenging, it stretched my mind and gave me something other than pregnancy and babies – or the lack of them – to think about. In September 1987, I became a first-year student on a single honours Sociology degree in a Midlands Polytechnic (now University). The decision to begin a degree was balanced against my desire to get pregnant but my husband encouraged me to go, saying that if I did I might get both of the things I then wanted – a baby and a degree – but if I did not go I might end up with nothing.

Although I got my degree and, a few years later, a PhD I have never, to my knowledge, been pregnant since that first time. My first marriage ended in my final undergraduate year, not solely because of our different views on pursuing parenthood, although inevitably this led to some unhappiness for both of us. My subsequent relationship with a man with two children earned me the status of step-mother, resulting in complex experiences and emotional responses for which I have no space here. My reflection on my miscarriage and subsequent 'infertility' continues. For my dissertation in the final year of my undergraduate degree I focused on experiences of miscarriage and in my doctoral research explored the social, emotional and medical experience of 'infertility' and 'involuntary childlessness'. From my own experiences I felt that pregnancy loss and non-motherhood were both misunderstood and under-researched and I've come across many others who feel the same; women (and men) who have had experiences more distressing than mine, individuals whose reproductive 'failures' dominate their lives. However, although it is important to highlight the structural factors that negatively impact on the identities and lives of those who experience miscarriage and 'infertility', it is also important to acknowledge individual differences, adjustments and adaptations. For some, reproductive loss and non-parenthood is less significant or something that they deal with and leave behind. Now self-defining as more (biologically) 'voluntarily childless' than 'involuntarily childless' I credit this shift in part to the opportunities my academic endeavours have given me for detailed reflection on my own experience and those of similar others, an opportunity that most people do not have. So this experience, alongside the continued support of those close to me and my relationship with my step-sons and the children of close friends, has been instrumental in a much more confident self-identity not dependent on biological motherhood.

62
A Family's Experience of Autopsy
Josie Hughes

Several years ago my Gran fell and broke her hip, and following several weeks in a convalescence home, she was allowed back home to the house she lived in with my step-grandad. Part of her physiotherapy was to get up and walk around the house every hour or so with the aid of a walking frame. One evening whilst she was having her walk my grandad heard a bang from the kitchen, and when he went in to her, she had fallen and hit her head and was unconscious. She was rushed into hospital

We have quite a dispersed family, with my dad living in the USA, my brother living in Canada, me living in the south of England, and my uncle and his family in the north. After her fall the England-based members of the family congregated at my Gran's bedside, taking it in turns to stay with her for the first 24 hours, as the medical staff didn't think she'd survive any longer than that. However, eventually we all began to return to our lives as the hospital felt she could go on indefinitely having survived initially, whilst all the time remaining unconscious.

When my Gran finally died only a few days later, she was alone in the hospital. My dad took this quite hard as his father had died alone in hospital in the middle of the night and dad had felt guilty about it at the time. And so he had asked me to make sure Gran wasn't left alone to die and I felt so terribly guilty that she had. My step-grandad was also struggling, as not only had he left her alone to die, but he hadn't been able to prevent her from falling – he felt that if he'd been watching her she wouldn't have fallen, and felt it was all his fault.

The day after my Gran died we were informed that she would have to undergo a post-mortem as the cause of death was unclear. By this point, I was back at home in the south of England, my dad had not yet arrived from the USA and my uncle had returned home, leaving my step-grandad to liaise with the hospital and doctors. This meant that all the information relating to the cause of death and the accident came second-hand via my step-grandad and so wasn't always as clear as it could have been had we been there to talk to the doctors ourselves. My uncle subsequently called the hospital for further clarification about the post-mortem, but was told it was 'standard procedure' in the event of an unexpected death. As we were all rather shocked by her death we didn't feel able to push the hospital for further details. With hindsight it was irrational, but at the time we felt that my step-grandad was being accused of hurting her, which, coupled with all our feelings of guilt around her death, made things very difficult and probably made us very uncooperative as a family.

I think we went into 'protect' mode and my uncle, who took over the liaison with the hospital, was very guarded in any information he gave them as he felt he didn't want to get my step-grandad into any 'trouble'. I think if we'd had the process of post-mortem explained more clearly at the outset and had understood that it was to find out exactly what happened and wasn't a case of placing blame, we would have found the ordeal much less painful as a family. Additionally, we would have been more willing to engage in a dialogue with the hospital and would have felt we could have asked them questions, which at the time we didn't feel comfortable doing in case it lead to any blame being placed. Again, it all seems very irrational now, but at the time we were dealing with our personal feelings over the loss of my Gran and the shock that it had happened when she had been recovering from a broken hip. There were also internal family politics (between my dad, his wife and two ex-wives – one of whom is my mum) – as to which wife would attend the funeral, and whether my half-sister – (from my dad's second marriage) would attend. All of this made the whole experience particularly stressful for me.

We received the results of the post-mortem after about a week. At the time it felt much longer, since events were suspended and we couldn't start to do the practical things like set the date for the funeral. My uncle was liaising with the hospital, so again the information I received was second-hand, but he said that the hospital had called him with the results. It turned out that she'd had a massive stroke, which had caused her fall, and it was this that had caused her eventual death; the fall was incidental. This meant that even if my step-grandad had been in the room with her it was likely to have still happened and she would have more than likely have died anyway.

When we got the results, there was a sense of relief that it was all over and that there wasn't anything my step-grandad could have done. My step-grandad was especially upset that she'd had to go through what he said he felt was the indignity of a post-mortem. My Gran had spent the latter years of her life in and out of hospital, mainly as a day patient, with my step-grandad accompanying her, and they had built up a very friendly relationship with a lot of the nursing staff. He said he felt as if some of the dignity she had always managed to preserve in the hospital had been taken away from her. My dad and I were upset about the thought of her being laid open and examined, I think we both felt, again irrationally, that she was somehow being violated and should have been left in peace. Gran was always very independent and proud, and it saddened me to think of a stranger cutting her open.

Despite all these feelings, in the long run having the post-mortem helped resolve a lot of the feelings of guilt my step-grandad had around her death. Additionally, a lot of what happened seems perfectly normal and rational looking back. I think that at the time there was so much emotion involved, it all seemed to be happening at a distance, and I was trying to mediate between my dad's immediate family so that everything seemed to be blown out of proportion. With hindsight, I think my Gran would probably have enjoyed it all – she always was a drama queen and didn't approve of my dad's third wife, so I think the thought of people arguing about who could come to her funeral, plus people worrying about how she died, would have rather appealed to her.

63
The First Death: A Student's Experience

Joyce Cavaye

Nothing prepares you for death. It was 1974 and I had been on my first ward for only two weeks when I had my first encounter with death. I remember feeling fear and embarrassment. Fear, because I hadn't seen a dead body before, and embarrassment at my own emotions. As a student nurse I had been schooled to keep my emotions under control. I had not yet developed the interpersonal skills that would later make this aspect of work more manageable. The death of Jane was a significant milestone in my nursing career – a time when the life-and-death nature of nursing and the realities of the job confronted me.

Jane (aged 78) had been admitted to the ward after falling at home. She had subsequently developed a chest infection and a deep vein thrombosis (DVT). She was a gentle, quiet, undemanding lady whose blue eyes filled with unshed tears as she surveyed her surroundings with a puzzled expression. It was as if she couldn't quite fathom out how she had come to be here in this ward surrounded by other ill people. During her time in the ward Jane was treated with antibiotics, prophylactic heparin and physiotherapy. She was expected to make a full recovery and return home.

Unknown to me, Jane's condition deteriorated as she developed pneumonia, her frail body too weak to fight the infection. Returning to the ward after my days off, I was surprised to see the curtains drawn round her bed which was now placed by the nurses' station. Her two daughters were sitting with her, holding her hands and speaking softly to her. They had been keeping a vigil for two days but were tired and needed a rest themselves. Jane went quietly in the early evening, shortly after her daughters had gone home and just before evening visiting.

As the most junior student on duty, I was assigned to 'do the body', arrange for the porter to remove it, and return this particular corner of the ward to rights. The instructions had been conveyed to me by the ward sister, an imposing figure whose brusque no-nonsense tone of voice brooked no argument. But, 'Where would I start?' 'What would I do?' I wondered as I gathered together the equipment usually required for a bed bath. I was nervous, scared and hesitant. Evelyn, a mature, experienced and sympathetic auxiliary nurse came to my rescue. She had seen the look of horror on my face and offered to help. Evelyn's advice was 'Pretend she's just sleeping, then it's easier to deal with'. This was said before we stepped behind the curtains!

Accompanied by Evelyn, I moved behind the curtains and looked at the body lying on the bed. All the ward sounds disappeared, all sense of panic evaporated – there was an atmosphere of absolute quiet calm. Gone was Jane, the bright-eyed, articulate and gracious lady; in her place was the pale, peaceful and serene face of a sleeping stranger. I didn't recognise the person she had been or had become. I had developed a good rapport with Jane and found much to chat with her about. She always had something to say and fascinating stories to tell about her life living in the Far East. But this body lying on the bed exposed to our stares wasn't Jane.

I remember vividly the sense of shock and fear I felt. Shock that Jane had deteriorated and died so quickly – she seemed too bright and alert for that to have happened. Fear that I was facing the unknown and wasn't sure how to react to a dead body. I was scared and ashamed of my feelings – my hands were as cold, stiff and awkward as the body lying still on the bed. In death Jane had simply become a body to be washed – another routine task was how Evelyn said we should regard it. A routine task that was carried out with almost indecent haste as Evelyn issued a continuous stream of instructions which I carried out as quietly and efficiently as possible. There was very little conversation between us.

As the ward doors opened for evening visitors, a sudden blast of cold air stirred the curtains around the bed and sent a chill down my spine. I checked Evelyn's reaction – nothing, she was quietly concentrating on the task in hand. I told myself not to be so fanciful, that the chill had nothing to do with death or the darkness outside at this time of night, it was just coincidence. But I was still scared. Scared enough to follow Evelyn out into the corridor and stay beside her as she phoned for the porters, rather than be left on my own with a dead body. Some nurse I was going to make if I couldn't deal with death!

Jane was left there behind the curtains – an anonymous body wrapped up in a sheet waiting for the porters to remove to her to the mortuary. Once visiting hour was over, we closed the curtains round all the beds in the ward. I tried to ignore the questions from patients who wanted to know why the curtains were being closed. Despite my silence, it didn't take long for the reason to be whispered from bed to bed. But we had at least to try and hide the reality of death from other patients. They couldn't be upset by the knowledge that someone had died. Even in hospitals there is a limit to what the public sees or is allowed to see or know.

The last task that I was charged with before the night shift came on was giving patients a hot drink. Apart from asking what they would prefer, tea, coffee, Horlicks or hot chocolate, I couldn't talk to patients. My reticence was noticed but accepted without comment. I found myself carrying out my duties automatically and letting my colleague do all the talking. I had nothing to say – no comments or observations to make. I was still too busy coming to terms with my first experience of death.

Rationalising death

Why was Jane's death so difficult for me to deal with? One reason was perhaps because death had not often been encountered in my day-to-day life. Nor was death a frequent topic of discussion, and until now I had little to do with death. Although my grandmother and brother had both died, I had been considered too young to attend their funerals. I came from a family where emotions and grief were dealt with in private and not discussed openly.

Another reason relates to feelings of competence. When I trained as a nurse, it was important for nurses to feel competent and convey a sense of being in control of their emotions and a clinical situation. Indeed, there was an expectation that students and nurses in general would learn to control their emotions. Such emotional control was regarded as part of a nurse's professional demeanour. A characteristic of a 'good' nurse was the ability to hide emotional reactions and to cultivate an air of emotional detachment, to professionally distance oneself from one's work. To be seen as being upset by the death of a patient was deemed to be unprofessional and you were therefore a 'bad' nurse. In the ward I had tried to be a good nurse by distancing myself and thinking of Jane as simply a body, an anonymous being. I deliberately overlooked our previous relationship, for to admit to that would open the floodgates of emotion. At home that night I allowed the tears to come, but whether they were for Jane or myself I was never very sure.

After my first experience of death, dealing with others became much easier over time. But so deeply was the virtue of emotional distance instilled in me that even 20 years later I continued to feel guilty and embarrassed by my emotions as I cried, not for the first time either, over the death of a patient – and there were many of them in the years I worked as a community nurse. Did this lack of emotional detachment mean that I was unprofessional? Did it make me a 'bad' nurse?

The role of education

The death of a patient is an experience that most nursing students will face. Yet my nurse training included very little teaching about death, dying and bereavement; it was mainly ward-based experiential learning. Since then there have been significant developments in both nurse education and end-of-life care. Nurse education is now diploma or degree based, with a more holistic approach to patient care. End-of-life care is no longer restricted to patients with cancer but has been extended to those with other chronic illnesses. Do these developments mean that nurses today are more adequately prepared to deal with death?

It would seem that they are not. Student nurses today continue to receive little training on how to deal with death, irrespective of whether they are undertaking a nursing diploma or degree. There is also little information on death and dying in undergraduate nursing textbooks. Education about death and dying is constructed as a specialist area, and mainly confined to post-basic and postgraduate courses which are taken by experienced nurses. The educational needs of nurses working with dying patients have to be addressed in pre- *and* post-registration education. Otherwise, how can we ever adequately prepare nurses to deal with death?

64
Death in Iceland, Hidden and Revealed

Arnar Árnason

I was fourteen, maybe fifteen. I had gone with my father to see a family friend in the small village I grew up in. We were hoping to borrow a trailer to take skidoos up to the mountains. Only, when we came to the house we noticed something that made us stop. In the garden in front of the house, the Icelandic flag was flying, half mast.

It has been the custom in Iceland for some time – in particular in the small rural communities where just about everyone knows everyone else – to fly the flag like this to mark the death of relatives. The flag is flown again on the morning of the day of the funeral, raised to the celebratory full mast once the funeral is over and the deceased has (hopefully) entered Heaven.

We knew, of course, that living with our friend and his family was his elderly mother. Had something happened to her, we wondered. For ten, fifteen minutes my father and I waited in the car, debating with ourselves whether to risk intruding on our friends' grief. Then again, we thought, the flag might be for some other more distant relative in the village. Eventually, we made our minds up and rang the bell. We were maybe ever so slightly spooked, but mainly relieved when the mother opened the door. Having borrowed the trailer we mentioned the flag to our friend, and asked him who had died. 'No one,' he said, 'it's Good Friday' ('Long Friday' literally in Icelandic, which seems a more appropriate name to me), and it is traditional to fly the flag half mast on this day. Then we told our friend about our hesitation, our fear for his mother, and everybody had a good laugh.

About two years ago the idea was put forward in an ever so slightly bigger village than the one I grew up in, to ban this flying of flags around deaths and funerals. The practice, it was said, is morbid, depressing. The building of a much debated bridge some twenty-five years ago means that the main road from Reykjavík to the North of Iceland now runs right through the middle of the village. In that time it has become a very popular place for travellers to stop and take refreshments. The surroundings are beautiful and the area historic. One of the most colourful heroes of the Icelandic Sagas lived there. It was suggested that the morbidity of death might discourage people from stopping, depress their desire to shop and consume. More recently, further road works mean that the village in question is now not much more than an hour's drive to or from Reykjavík, the starting point or destination of most journeys coming through. Maybe travellers will start to feel less inclined to stop when, whether coming or going, it is only a question of an hour.

At about the same time as it was being suggested that morbid flag-flying be banished from villages in Iceland, posters, often adorned with starkly black crosses, started to appear on bridges and other structures in Reykjavík, asking car drivers and their passengers such things as: Will you return home safely? Are you hurrying towards eternity? Will today be the last day you overtake? (playing on the fact that to overtake and to get up, *fara fram úr*, is the same phrase in Icelandic). The posters appeared just before what is traditionally a very busy weekend of travelling in Iceland. While some people were rather disturbed and read them initially as a threat, their aim is of course to enhance road safety and reduce traffic accidents. Their sentiments, indeed some of the actual phrases, have been publicised. Their authors and sponsors are public institutions of various sorts that are directly responsible for road safety, like the Road Traffic Directorate, or private enterprises whose interests are served by greater road safety, like insurance companies.

Recent years have seen the emergence, indeed proliferation, of roadside memorials in Iceland. Most often small white crosses, they are publicly placed but private in that the victim remains unnamed. Thus they are unlike the crosses in graveyards, which they resemble, even as, like their graveyard counterparts, many of them are clearly visited regularly.

I find in this an intriguing paradox. On the one hand is the idea – even if it was only an idea – to banish the public proclamation of death and mortality. On the other hand is the very public, even aggressive, reminder of mortality and the possibility of death. And the paradox reminds me that death in Iceland is never simply personal and private. A sense of loss and redemption has pervaded many accounts of Icelandic history. As more and more people live in the relative anonymity of the city (and in Iceland it is still very much relative), the flying of the flag to announce death loses some of its meaning. But still flags are conspicuous by their presence in mortuary rites in Iceland. And individual stories of loss and redemption can help to foster the notion of the nation as a community, even though that has to be increasingly imagined. The threat of extinction – of the nation, its language, heritage and culture – has been a pervasive element of many political debates in Iceland. Evoking this element helps to turn the effort of reducing the number of fatal accidents on the roads into a project that is both individual and national, private and public.

65
My Floral Tribute

Maxine Birch

When Kevin was dying, our home suddenly became a pilgrimage for his many friends and family. We could easily receive more than six different visits, with varying numbers of visitors, each day. This occurred for about three months. When groups of people were assembled I often felt like I was left jostling for some sort of position or recognition. My relationship with Kevin was complex and hard to describe succinctly. We could tick certain relationship type categories but not others. Yes, we had been together for ten years, but we had only formally 'lived together' for one year. We both had our own families that we brought together in varying combinations. We engaged with the usual parenting roles, but for different children from different marriages. Plus we were exploring a brand new joint role of being a granddad and extra 'granny'. This complex web of family relationships felt inclusive, sometimes creating great tensions and at other times building great friendships. Sharing these complex family relationships was more often than not a rewarding experience, but the words used to describe these shared family relationships were limited: I was not a step-mother, but I was more than a friend. At the end of the day this lack of words meant that my son was not Kevin's son, and this delineated 'my family' from 'his family'. During this time of impending loss, this was a distinction that appeared to me to achieve a greater significance.

When Kevin's dying combined with the many visitors, the experience of 'our family' became harder and harder to negotiate. I no longer knew where I was in his life and as his life was ending the sense of having a shared one was lost. He was my partner but not quite my husband. He was a key part of my children's lives but did not fulfil the more familiar role of step-father or uncle. Who I was within his family I could never fathom. We didn't even possess a joint mortgage but were designated co-owners. I was suddenly the person who had been with him only for a small part of his life. Irrespective of how frequent or infrequent the contact had previously been between Kevin and his brothers and sisters, suddenly the claim for being a member of Kevin's childhood family gained increasing importance. His many friends would also visit and make similar claims for being a more essential part of his past. This was supported by tales of shared histories during critical periods, with childhood memories as the most seductive. There is nothing wrong with this, and I know that in similar circumstances I would make the same demands to acknowledge my shared history with my siblings and friends. In this instance, most importantly, I needed to know where I fitted within Kevin's life. Against these stories of shared past experiences, my experiences of trying to be together became less tangible. As I managed Kevin's dying on a daily basis, I realised the importance of social recognition. I wanted a formal role, a wife, a relative, not just the resident carer or some other 'girlfriend'. After Kevin's death these feelings took on much significance for me and became a source of further distress. This was when I found so much solace in flowers.

Flowers and death are inseparable for me. My mother always told me that she could smell lilies when death was threatening someone we knew. I lost my mother in my twenties; she was

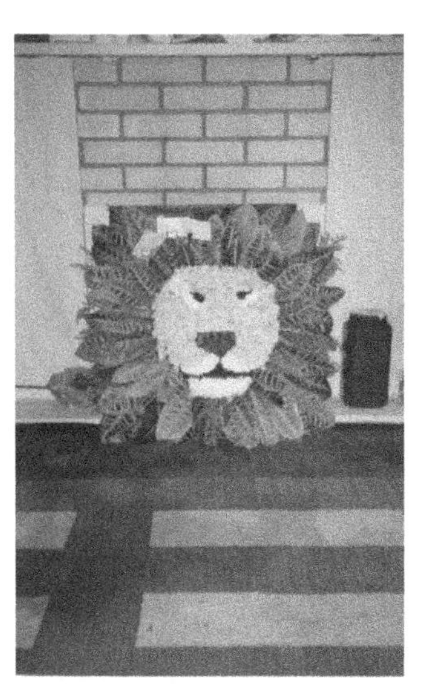

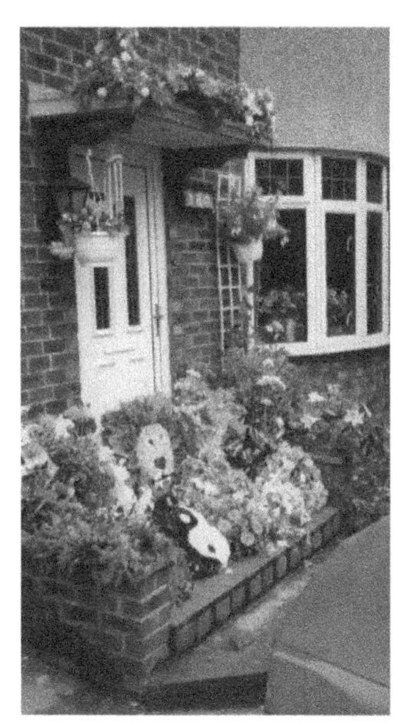

only 58. My mother had lost her mother at a similar age, and this was connected to her assertions about lilies and death. Added to this foundation was my mother's love of flowers. My mother was a florist. She was also part of the church flower rota. Hence following the sudden death of my mother it felt very natural to go overboard with the flowers. My sister and I decorated the church with so many flowers that some friends and acquaintances commented that our display was more suitable for a wedding, not a funeral. So it was no surprise to me that after Kevin's death I turned to flowers once again.

I requested flowers and I was surrounded by flowers from the day of the funeral to several weeks later when the last one rotted on my front door step. Flowers arrived in all shapes and sizes: from formal tributes usually seen at funerals; large bouquets of flowers that I promptly placed in vases around the house; to specific symbols, made from flower petals, which represented Kevin's personality. I don't know what spurred me to bring the flowers home from the crematorium, but I did. I placed them all around the front door. This was the front door of the house where Kevin and I had tried, for a brief time, to build a future together. This floral display stopped the postman delivering the mail, it stopped visitors from ringing the doorbell. The flowers denoted the end of the pilgrimage. Only those who are close to me would confidently come round to the backdoor. It filled the house with a wonderful smell from dawn to dusk. Local people would stand and stare. Distant neighbours were in no doubt about what had happened in my household. Part of accepting Kevin's death was to try to bring together the complex feelings of loss – for the partnership that I felt was never recognised or fully achieved, and for the person he was. This floral tribute helped these complex feelings to exist more comfortably together. The flowers outside my door became my public recognition for my personal loss. Today the photographs can still bring me back in touch with a sense of finding myself within all this chaos.

66
Silenced Endings: Death, Dying and Learning Disabilities

Stuart Todd

[...]

Background

The study reported here was concerned with the deaths of people with learning disabilities, with the dying phase of a person's life and how support was provided at such times and, indeed, beyond. It describes how dying is managed in learning disability settings, places that are typically characterized as places of 'living'. It examines the perspectives of parents about what it means to lose a child with learning disabilities. Finally it also examines the ways in which people with learning disabilities themselves looked at death. [...]

Death counts. It counts in the way individuals have death anxieties. It counts for relatives and friends who have to deal with the loss of a loved one. It counts for many services who will have to provide end-of-life support to people who are dying. It counts socially since society has to continue around, as well as accommodate to, death. However, not all deaths count in the same way, and the silence that surrounds death, dying and learning disability is of some concern. Social inequalities are not washed away at the end of life. Instead they persist and outlive us. Thus, since we know the difference being labelled as having a learning disability can make to a person's life, it also seems pertinent to ask, "What difference does it make to the matters of dying and of death?" Some might view such a question as inappropriate and wasteful! After all, there remain so many features of a person's life that are restricted that to focus on death and dying can only be seen as distractions from the real business and challenge of living. However, if we were to stop and say, "Death doesn't count here! We are not interested in how people with learning disabilities die or how people grieve for them after their death!" What would such an answer mean? That we do not value the lives of people with learning disabilities? Life and death are inseparable! They cannot be teased and kept apart. To study one is to understand the other. Dying, death and bereavement will be given a particular shape by 'learning disability' and it is important to understand its influence at the end of life.

[...]

Data were obtained on 17 deaths that had taken place in supported living settings. Interviews were also held with 14 bereaved parents of people with learning disabilities. Finally, 12 people with

---

Stuart Todd, 'Silenced endings: Death, dying and learning disabilities', a summary report of a research study funded by the Henry Smith Charity, Welsh Centre for Learning Disabilities, Cardiff University. Reproduced by kind permission of the author.

learning disabilities were interviewed about their own experiences and perspectives about death. All interviews were semi-structured so as to allow people to talk fully about their experiences.

[...]

Findings

Such lonely endings: the experiences of bereaved parents

For many parents, the death of a child with learning disabilities was largely unexpected. Although some parents had been told that their children might have shorter lives, the age when death might come was unknown. For some other parents, the death of their child had never been anticipated. Thus for many bereaved parents, the death of their child came 'out-of-the-blue':

> We had been on holiday and Gerry was in respite. We found out two days after his death. Our son was home. He was nineteen and had to do the formalities. I never thought when I said good bye to him on the Monday that was to be the last time. He'd never been ill.

In the days after the death of their child, and in particular, after the funeral, parents found that the world with which they had been a central part of for many years was withdrawing. In some cases, this seemed to be done with haste and without much sensitivity, as the following examples below indicate:

> There was no offer of support from them (social services). I was told on the day of her funeral that I wouldn't be seeing anyone again.

> Everything stopped. I'd known them for years (services) – they knew me – but it all stopped as soon as she died!

Nearly all parents reported that they had wanted some on-going contact with services and their support needs had not ended with the death of their child. Some parents had managed to keep in contact with other parents of children with disabilities. They reported that the people in this 'world' understood their loss or in a way that others were unable to. For other parents who did not manage to have on-going contact with other people who had some insight into 'learning disability', the time after the death of their child was lonely and confusing. Certainly, the withdrawal of this specialist world was felt to be untimely. All families described their loss as profound, a feeling they felt not everyone understood, as the following comment from one mother makes abundantly clear:

> Freedom's not all it's cracked up to be! I miss her. The touch of her. She was full of life and she was my life! I'd do the housework around her, I did everything around her. It was my whole life. All that pain from the day she was born 'til the day she died? I wouldn't want to be without it. I still want her back. A part of me went with her! I don't know what to do with myself.

What many parents reported was a lack of emotional support in their own networks to help them through and adjust to their loss. Indeed rather than finding a sympathetic community, parents found that there was a tendency in others to transform their loss into a 'gain' or a 'relief':

> My family deep down thought it was a blessing.

The feelings of many parents did not seem to be acknowledged by others and to such an extent that the bereavement experience was privatised:

> When you talk about it – you can talk about it – but you feel you're not allowed to show how you feel. That you're just supposed to get on with it. It's like you're sitting on an emotional volcano! I don't think anybody understands at all!

The bereavement experiences of parents can be described as an example of 'disenfranchised grief'. That is a from of grief that is seldom recognized or supported, when, in turn, the individual with a learning disability is grieved over. It refers to a difficult to bear form of grief, of which there were three dimensions. To begin with there was a sense that others did not see the relationship between parent and child as 'real'. Parents felt that if the death related to their non-disabled child, the reaction of others would have been different:

> I didn't feel that they understood. No-one to guide me through it. If Rachel had been her sister the loss would have been as devastating but people would've understood. It was like I had to say, 'But Rachel is my daughter too'!

The second dimension relates to the scope of loss. The loss of a child was severely felt, however as mothers in particular stated, it also involved the loss of a way of life. Many mothers had given up work and over time, social contacts, to look after their son or daughter with learning disabilities. Research clearly supports this view and that services provide little scope for parents to carry on with life as they had before. Thus when a child with a learning disability dies, there is no world for a parent to return to. The world of learning disability stops and the world with which they used to interact prior to the birth of their child is also no longer there. It is, then a multiple loss which involves the child, communities and a sense of identity:

> I still struggle to make sense of things. For some people, well they can go back even if they hurt. I couldn't! There was nothing there for me. Just a void. Everything was completely gone. I had empty hours and a huge hole in my heart.

Finally, as indicated above the loss parents have experienced is not disregarded or insignificant, it is seen by some as a positive gain!

> Some people thought it must be a relief. It's not the way it was. It was never that to me! To me it was just loss! Just grief!
>
> [...]

Hidden dying: the death views of people with learning disabilities

The final group of people from whom data were obtained were people with learning disabilities themselves. It has been argued that there are three fundamental secrets we keep from people with learning disabilities. Sex and disability are two of these. Death is said to be the third and most painful secret. Although death might be considered to be a secret, it as an aspect of life that people in the study had experienced. During my conversations with people, there was an eagerness to talk about death. Many of them had experienced the loss of someone they loved or cared for. These were, for example, parents, siblings, children, grandparents or friends. Death was not something that only happened to some people. It happened to everyone. There was a recognition of the universality and irreversibility of death:

> Everyone will die one day. And when you're dead, you're dead.

Everyone who had experienced a death had taken part in death rituals, for example, viewing the body and/or funerals. People were also able to talk about how they would prefer to die and how their bodies should be disposed of:

> I'd like to be buried for my family. My parents could still visit me. It would be like I could be there for them. If you're cremated you're just gone!

However, for all the people I spoke to the death of a loved one seemed to have been unexpected. Clearly, in some cases this was the case. However, in others it seemed that the death of an individual had only been unexpected to the person with a learning disability. Some deaths were described that would surely have been preceded by a period of dying. However, the dying phase was one that was hidden from them. Few people had a view of dying that was anything other than sudden and peaceful. Predictable death after a period of illness was less well recognised. One man said of the death of his mother:

> My mam passed away see. I think she'd been ill for a long time. But I never knew she was going to die. She always talked to me. She's gone now. I don't know how she died. She never said 'Goodbye'. My dad never speaks about it.

The idea that one could be dying and living at the same time was a difficult concept to explain. For most people dying implied close to death and weakness. Some had a view of dying that was chiefly influenced by television dramas. Here the imagery of machines keeping people alive was prevalent:

> The first thing I'd do would be to get a second opinion. But if I wasn't getting better and I was getting worse. I wouldn't want it. I'd tell my mum and dad to switch it off. Just let me go!

People were asked how they would like to be remembered or what impact their deaths would have on others. Almost everyone said they would like to be remembered as 'happy'. However, when they were asked who would remember them, participants with parents mentioned only their parents. This limited imagined community of mourners reflects perhaps a limited social network. For those whose parents had already died, there were few other possible mourners. Reference might be made to a 'brother' or 'sister'. For one person, it would be the people in the office where he worked two days a week. He remarked:

> The people I work with. They wouldn't have anyone to empty the bins in their offices. They'd be thinking about me because they'd be missing me. I do my work well. The bins, the paper and the bags. I take them out to a wheelie bin. They wouldn't have anybody do that if I died.
>
> […]

Part VI

Reflecting on Traumatic Death, Mass Death and Disaster

Introduction

Sarah Earle and Carol Komaromy

Most of the pieces in Part V explore the feelings and experiences of individuals following the death of someone close. While these experiences share some similarities, and indeed each death carries a traumatic dimension for many people, the experiences of people bereaved following mass death and disaster bears unique features, and so they have been given a place of their own here in Part VI.

This part begins with two pieces, both of which focus on the aftermath following the Asian Tsunami of 26 December 2004. The first of these, which has been specially commissioned for this volume, is written by Claire Wijayatilake, a teacher living and working in Sri Lanka, and it focuses on the experiences of children and their families. Making sense of the loss of so many people of all ages carries its own challenges for bereaved survivors. The second, by Prathap Tharyan, focuses on the importance of ritual in managing grief in India following the Tsunami. The role of ritual at the time of loss has many different forms, and while it has changed over time and varies between cultures it remains an enduring coping mechanism after death. In the next contribution, Lesley Moreland also focuses on the issue of grief and bereavement as she describes the murder of her daughter Ruth, and provides a powerful insight into the immediate effects of traumatic death. Of course, longer term, mass death and disaster can have significant consequences for survivors and those who have been bereaved. In another piece specially commissioned for this volume, Carol Komaromy offers personal reflections on the death of her father and, in particular, on the continuing impact of what he witnessed at the Nazi concentration camp at Belsen in 1945, not just on him but on his children too. The next piece has been written by members of *Disaster Action*, a charity set up and run by people who have either survived disaster or been bereaved by an event. This piece, which highlights the 'huge range of reactions', mirrors and emphasises the variety and diversity of feelings and experiences following mass death and disaster, which can be seen in the selection of examples presented in this part of the book.

The next three contributions focus specifically on the feelings and experiences of individuals professionally involved in caring for people following traumatic death, mass death and disaster. In the first of these three pieces, Tom Heller, a GP, offers personal and professional reflections on his involvement in the disaster on 15 April 1989 at the football grounds in Hillsborough, showing that all of those involved, even those carrying the brief of professional support, are affected by such events. Since Hillsborough, the traumatic effects on carers have been recognised and the expectations of coping reframed and renegotiated. Next, in a piece commissioned for this volume, Patricia Wiltshire describes her work as a forensic ecologist, exploring the ways in which she manages this role. In the last of these three pieces, Lucy Easthope explores her experiences of returning personal property after death and disaster.

In the final piece in Part VI, Anne Eyre, a crisis management consultant, reflects on the impact of sudden mass death following the attacks on the World Trade Centre in New York on 11 September 2001. Drawing on first-hand accounts from fire-fighters and others, Anne Eyre asks 'what can we learn from this?' Anne's work in this area stemmed from her personal experience of being a football spectator at the fated Hillsborough disaster.

67

When the Tsunami Hit Sri Lanka

Claire Wijayatilake

At least one-third of the 232,000 people who were killed or are still missing across a dozen Indian Ocean nations hit by the 26 December 2004 tsunami were children. The hundreds of thousands who survived are coping with the loss of family members, teachers and friends. Life in tsunami-hit areas will probably never be the same again. Even those officially 'unaffected' are certainly not without scars, which remain two and a half years on. I was in Sri Lanka on the ill-fated day, not in an affected area, thankfully, but I can vouch for the fact that the children all over the island were affected in so many ways. But it is those children who were directly affected through the loss of their homes and loved ones whose scars remain most vivid.

When the tsunami hit Sri Lanka at around 9.25 a.m., 6-year-old Tharuka* was enjoying a day at the beach with his parents, 10-year-old sister Seneli, and several aunts, uncles and cousins. It was a Poya (full-moon) day, a holiday for Buddhists, and the beach at Hambantota on the south coast was full of families relaxing at this popular holiday resort.

When the water level started to rise, Tharuka's family, like so many others, had no idea what was happening, but ran for cover towards the nearby salt drying pits; instead of escaping the water, they met the sea coming towards them on the other side of the pits. Tharuka grabbed onto a log, which saved his life, but he saw his sister and one of his aunts disappear beneath the waves. Clinging on for dear life, the little boy was washed up inside one of the salt pits, and spent two days surrounded by dead bodies, waiting for rescue. Perhaps it was a self-protection mechanism that made him believe that the dead were just sleeping. He only felt sad for a deer, which lay dead beside him.

Tharuka was found by a man who had come looking among the dead for his own loved ones, and he was taken to hospital by Air Force personnel in charge of the rescue operation. One of the airmen was later to tell Tharuka's parents that the terrified child had been unable to stop talking – he spoke of the speech he was going to give to welcome the new students to his school in January, and the coloured pens he had received as a gift from his aunt the day before the disaster – anything and everything except the horrors he had lived through in the last few days.

Meanwhile, Tharuka's distraught parents were searching through the truckloads of bodies arriving at the hospitals for their missing son, daughter and other relatives. Finally they discovered Seneli's body, lying on the floor of a hospital because the morgue was full. They buried her quickly along with two of her aunts and her 3-year-old cousin. The family's servant girl, who Tharuka adored, also died in the tragedy.

---

*All of the children's names have been changed.

The following day, Tharuka's parents finally discovered their little boy at a hospital. He didn't speak of Seneli or the aunt he saw drowning or of any of the horrors he had witnessed. He didn't talk about his feelings, which must have been overwhelming. Instead, he complained to his mother that no-one had given him anything to eat and asked for food.

The couple got ready to take their son home, but Tharuka refused to leave the hospital without Seneli. He was convinced she was alive and 'lost' somewhere as he had been. The desperate parents finally told their son his sister had gone to Australia to their aunt as she needed treatment there. I have noticed that Sri Lankan parents often avoid telling children about deaths or serious illnesses in an attempt to spare their feelings, and Tharuka chose to believe the story in spite of evidence to the contrary. Newspaper reporters visited the family and asked them about Seneli's death. Tharuka told them they had got it wrong. During the seventh-day (after death) Buddhist rites for the dead members of the family, the monks mentioned Seneli's name along with those of the other victims. Tharuka told his mother the monks had made a mistake. When this brave little boy returned to school a month after the tragedy, his classmates teased him, saying 'you think your sister is in Australia but actually she's dead'.

The tsunami changed Tharuka's personality. From being a talkative and open little boy he became quiet and reserved. He refused to go near the sea or see pictures of it. When the family traveled to the south coast to give alms on the anniversary of the tragedy, he closed his eyes through Hambantota, refusing to look at the hotel where his young life had been shattered. He wouldn't look at pictures of Seneli or let anyone speak of her. He started to cry at the slightest provocation, had nightmares and refused to sleep without his parents at his side. From being a bright student, he lost interest in his school work and his grades went down. It's now two and a half years since the tragedy but there are no photos of Seneli in the family home and no-one speaks of her. It's the way they have chosen to cope.

While Tharuka's parents and grandmother have found strength in their Buddhist faith, which has deepened since the disaster, religion is not something Tharuka connects in any way with his ordeal. He doesn't talk about her being reborn or being in a better place. There is only one context in which he ever speaks of his sister. When another child, particularly a girl, does something wrong, Tharuka says 'My Akki (big sister) wouldn't do that. She's better than her.' Though Seneli was a normal child who had a normally acrimonious relationship with her little brother, he has idealized her in death.

We might assume that Tharuka felt guilty that he had lived while his sisters, aunts and little cousin died. He appears to be avoiding the guilt by rationalizing what happened. 'She (Seneli) ran the wrong way', he says. 'If she had run the same way as me, she would have lived.' It sounds callous, but is an explanation that has helped the confused boy to cope.

Tharuka appears to be back to normal now. He's studying well and his old personality has returned, but he still can't talk about what happened that day in December 2004.

My own children, especially the elder one, Anisha, who was 10 at the time, have, like all Sri Lankan children, been affected. Seneli was her teacher's granddaughter and the same age as her. She was acutely aware that, seeing her alive and well, had a profound effect on her teacher during the first year after the tsunami. Two children at Anisha's school died, which affected her greatly. For months, my daughter was plagued by nightmares, in which a 'ghost' plucked her from a chair in our living room and she never saw her family again. For my younger child, two and a half at the time, 'tsunami' became synonymous with 'monster' and she suffered generalized fears and insecurities. Both children went from adoring the beach to refusing to go near it for more than a year.

I was a teacher in Colombo at that time and found the children I taught very much affected by what had happened. They seemed profoundly unable to process the information they had received, either from direct experience or from stories and TV reports they had seen or heard. What struck me most was the number of inappropriate reactions I encountered among my students. When the topic was brought up, it was often met with jokes and nervous laughter. Although my first reaction was to tell them off, I later realized that their absolute unpreparedness for something of that magnitude caused them to revert to the comfortable, familiar mode of humour in order to avoid engagement with the horrors they should never have had to face.

Children in Sri Lanka are typically wonderful artists, and draw prolifically in a clearly identifiable style. After the tsunami, children's art changed; it became darker, with themes of destruction and death. Schools, counselors and the volunteers in the refugee camps realized early on that art was a useful outlet for the children's' emotions, and soon art supplies were requested from donors as much as food and water.

Colleagues from my school were amazed by the resilience of children in the camps when they visited them to run 'activity days'. Youngsters who had lost their whole families joined in the cricket, sing-songs and games. Our drama teacher ran 'drama therapy' courses in camps as another way of enabling affected children to express their experiences.

Two and a half years on, people are finally beginning to believe that another tsunami on the same scale is probably not just around the corner. The beaches are full of families enjoying the sand and sea. Children's art is full of life and colour again. But the shadow of 26 December 2004 is still over the children of Sri Lanka. Many have been relocated away from the areas where they lived before and are still suffering from the loss of the family breadwinner or caregiver. For the rest, the concept of 'tsunami' has entered their consciousness forever, as a kind of awareness of their own fragility, a realization that their lives, once so solid and certain, could be gone in an instant, swallowed up by a something as 'harmless' as a wave.

68

Traumatic Bereavement and the Asian Tsunami: Perspectives from Tamil Nadu, India

Prathap Tharyan

[...]

Overall, the tsunami killed more than 280,000 people, displaced more than one million and affected the lives of around five million more (WHO, 2005). India was less affected than Indonesia, Thailand or Sri Lanka, but over 2,000 km of the country's eastern coast bore the brunt of nature's fury, unprecedented in living memory. The district of Nagapattinam in Tamil Nadu accounted for more than 6,000 of the 8,000 dead, mostly women, children and the elderly. Over 5,000 people were reported missing and many are still unaccounted for.

[...]

The nature of bereavement in India

Grief is a private matter in most Western societies and the expression of grief is largely subdued and restricted to the funeral parlour and the privacy of one's home or the offices of a bereavement counsellor. This is consistent with the ethos of life in the West, where self-determination and privacy are cherished facts of life, as opposed to traditional practices in South Asian countries, where individual desires are subjugated by the dictates of common affiliations to families, communities, religious traditions, gender, and trans-generational roles. Interest in others' affairs is not seen as an invasion of privacy but rather as a connectedness, interdependence and involvement in the lives of important others. Consequently, grieving is a community affair and expressions of grief and mourning are loud and publicly demonstrated, funeral processions are as tumultuous as wedding processions, and there are well-delineated roles and social customs associated with grieving that are universally observed.

Prathap Tharyan, 'Traumatic bereavement and the Asian Tsunami: Perspectives from Tamil Nadu, India', extract taken with permission from an article originally published in *Bereavement Care* 2005; 24(2): 21–4.

The importance of rituals

The many rituals associated with death and bereavement in traditional Indian culture pertain to ancient notions of pollution and purification that ensure the repose of the departed soul (Kaltman and Bonanno, 2003). Our first visit to Nagapattinam coincided with one such ritual or *karyam* where prayers were said by priests for the departed and in most households that had suffered a loss, pictures of loved ones were placed before glowing lamps, incense, flowers and religious offerings. Such rituals allow survivors to confront their grief, bring families and communities together and help punctuate, and eventually set limits to, the process of grieving.

In one of the villages we visited, the administration had arranged a community memorial service for the children who lost their lives in the tsunami. Parents planted coconut saplings in memory of each of their lost children and this memorial will stand as a living reminder of the loss the village suffered, as well as a tribute to the compassion of an administration that used a novel method to share in the grief of a traumatised people.

Spiritual traditions and practices

Spiritual beliefs and practices are widespread in Indian culture and, though the fishermen of costal Tamil Nadu are not marked by particular religious practices that demarcate them from other communities, there is a widespread belief in the immutable soul or *atman*. There is also a common subscription to evil spirits, sorcery, the evil eye and other notions of spiritualism, existing in easy harmony with more modern notions of natural causation, concepts borrowed from the ancient ayurvedic tradition, and the western medical model of infectious diseases.

For many, the tsunami was seen as an act of nature, for others it was an act of a displeased god. Whatever their views on the cause, the near universal belief in the karmic cycle of birth and rebirth (where the *atman* returns to find abode in another, hopefully more pious or respected, life-form) could prevent some of the fears and concerns of those who believe in reward or retribution after death. However, I am unaware of any comparative study of the effects of these contrasting beliefs on the process of mourning, though empirical evidence indicates that even in Western societies, people who profess stronger spiritual beliefs seem to resolve their grief more rapidly and completely than do those with no spiritual beliefs (Walsh et al., 2002).

[...]

References

Kaltman S, Bonanno GA. Trauma and bereavement: examining the impact of sudden and violent deaths. *Journal of Anxiety Disorders* 2003; 17: 131–147.

Walsh K, King M, Jones, Tookman A, Blizard R. Spiritual beliefs may affect outcome of bereavement: prospective study. *British Medical Journal* 2002; 324: 1551.

World Health Organisation. Three months after the Indian Ocean earthquake-tsunami: health consequences and WHO's response. http://www.who.int/hac/crises/international/asia_tsunami/3months/en/index.html, posted 08/April/2005.

69

Ruth: Death by Murder

Lesley Moreland

As the New Year 1990 started our family life seemed to have entered on a new and welcome stage. Our eldest daughter had married happily and moved to Knebworth in 1988 when she was 24 and our youngest daughter, then 22, had moved to share a rented house with friends in Enfield in the same year.

I had left my job as Director of the Stillbirth and Neonatal Death Society (SANDS) early in 1989 and had taken a big leap into working freelance, partly as a management consultant in the voluntary sector and also starting a very small business in holding craft workshops. We felt, maybe somewhat smugly, pride in our daughters and that our relationship with them and with each other was strong and loving and life looked very good indeed.

On 2 February, just as we had finished eating our evening meal, the doorbell rang. What happened after that was like a nightmare except that it was real. The callers were police officers who came to let us know that our youngest daughter, Ruth, was dead. She had been murdered and a young man was held in custody. The police were and have remained very certain that he is the person who killed her. We had never heard his name before Ruth died. Her 24th birthday was on 6 February and we had been expecting to see her over the weekend.

My years at SANDS had given me a wider than average background in the theory of bereavement and a great deal of contact with people in the various stages of grieving. In some ways this was helpful, in others it seemed to hamper the free expression of feelings.

Forgiveness

The Greek philosopher Aristotle said that there was one loss from which a person could never recover, and that was the loss of a child. It struck too deeply, he thought, at the foundations of a life for there ever to be a chance of rebuilding.

Since Ruth died there has been a constant struggle to survive rather than become a victim of her loss. I have always been aware that the issue of forgiveness of the person who killed her would need to be faced but this was difficult to even begin as our family had never even heard the name of the young man who was charged with her murder until after her death. Many people asked how I felt about him and I found it impossible to answer, although I had no problem with how I felt about what he had done.

Ralph Hetherington wrote a commentary about forgiveness in *The Friend* in January 1991 which was published in the week before the trial of the young man charged with Ruth's

---

Lesley Moreland, 'Ruth: Death by murder', in Dickenson, Johnson, Samson Katz (eds), *Death, Dying and Bereavement*, 2nd edn. SAGE, 2000, pp. 376–8. Reproduced by kind permission of the publisher and author.

murder. The article considered whether repentance was a prerequisite for forgiveness and stressed the need to recognize the dangers of judging people who have harmed us. It seems to me that passing judgement on others is difficult partly because we cannot understand why someone has behaved in a way which has hurt us or those we love and partly because we have to recognize our own failings in our behaviour towards other people.

I was shocked that evidence given during the trial seemed to reveal no remorse or insight into the suffering caused to Ruth and all those who loved her. One of my nieces, who also attended the trial, said 'I needed to see that he was sorry and he wasn't'.

But life takes many unexpected turns. When the trial was over I contacted a friend who is a probation officer. It hadn't occurred to me that the young man would be sent to the prison where she works. With our agreement, she saw him and he asked that a message should be sent to us to say how sorry he was, how much he admired and respected Ruth and that she had always been very kind to him. I was also able to send a message to him in which I hoped that he would accept any help offered to him to help him understand why he had done what he had done, to use any opportunities to extend his skills and education and to resolve to use the rest of his life in positive ways both for himself and for others. However, I couldn't bring myself to send a message of forgiveness.

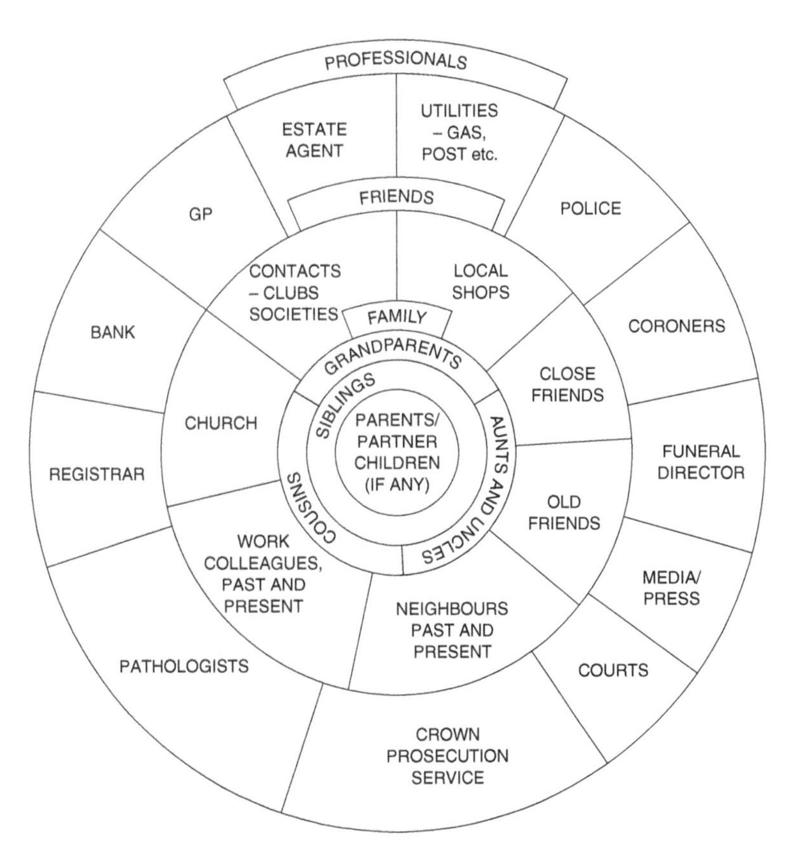

Figure: Circles of support. Based on work done by Birmingham and Surrey SANDS. 1987.

Those affected and involved in the aftermath of murder

A month after Ruth was murdered her employers held a gathering of her colleagues and many of the people who had attended the courses that she had arranged for women returners. The event was guided by a man who described those present in terms of having been affected by an 'earthquake' and spoke of those in Ruth's family as being at the 'epicentre'.

The illustrated Circles of Support is not intended to make distinctions between the depth of people's feelings – we were very aware that many who were involved professionally were also emotionally affected. Rather it is intended to give Victim Support volunteers a framework so that they can be aware of the numbers and kinds of people who are affected or involved in the aftermath of a murder.

Those included in the circle will vary with each murder. We were spared any direct press or media involvement; for other families this will be a major aspect.

Reference

Hetherington. R. (1991) 'Commentary'. *The Friend,* 149 (3): 67–8.

70

Reflections of Death: Continuing Memories

Carol Komaromy

My father was someone I was proud of. His humour was something I treasured most and he seemed to be able it use it to make light of difficult situations. Not only did he make us laugh with his pithy observations of life, he was also gentle and kind. However, he had an obsessive pre-occupation with safety and seemed to see danger in everything. For example, it was not unusual to get frequent calls at bedtime reminding me to lock my door, and to receive regular gifts of torches and even bolts to make the house more secure. I discovered that his fears that so irritated my sister and I were founded in a reality that terrible things do happen. Of course, by the time I realised this it was almost too late.

He was dying when he talked to me about Belsen. He had cancer and had taken on the appearance of a victim of starvation. He was pale, emaciated and had a piercing look of fear in his eyes. I had known about his experience for over ten years, when my nephew had interviewed him for a history project as part of his homework, but my dad had never talked to me about it and my mother had warned me off by saying, 'It is all too upsetting and something that should be forgotten'. He had witnessed Belsen in the first days of its discovery. Suddenly, it was urgent that he told me. I knew that this memory must be part of his reflections on life and I wanted to help him. He was being given pain relief for his physical pain, but I was worried about his emotional state. I did not want him to suffer in any way.

He and I agreed that he would talk to me about it and in preparation for our conversation he had written down his story. His writing was barely legible. My dad was born in Northern Ireland in 1921 and left school at 14. Even so, he was someone who barely attended school because he hated it so much. He was intelligent and uneducated, and the latter embarrassed him.

Here is part of what he told me: 'One day, following the big push forward after the D-day landings, we were camped in some woods and our commanding officer asked for volunteers to go into a camp nearby to take in water and some flour. John and I volunteered and I drove our truck down a dirt track to the camp that was hidden deep in the woods. There we saw terrible sights. I saw dead bodies on toilets; dead bodies in sheds piled 12 high and a young woman who looked eighty. The smell of the corpses was terrible. Starved and frightened people who surrounded us scrambled for water and begged us to take them with them. We did not know what to do; how to help these poor starving people. We gave them our rations and then John started to sing to them. He was Welsh and had a wonderful voice and as he sang smiles came upon their faces. When we left this small group of people gathered around us, they were smiling. We were only there for a few hours, but the nightmare of what I saw has stayed with me all my life. I cannot forget the sights I saw. We had many a bad experience but Belsen will always stay with me as my worst experience. When I think about it now the worst part is trying to understand how someone could do this to another human being; trying to understand that cruelty, but the sight is there every time I shut my eyes. I tried to forget but I can't.'

My father was totally without emotion as he told me the story. His most worrying concern was what had happened to those people and if they had managed to get 'home'.

I felt that I had to acknowledge what had happened and in my quest to ease his emotional pain I set out to find a survivor to let him know that it had been possible for people to survive. Indeed, that year was the anniversary of the liberation of Belsen and to commemorate the occasion a permanent exhibition was being installed in the Imperial War Museum. My partner helped me to trace a Jewish survivor's group. Through this Jewish group and to coincide with the unveiling of the exhibition, I was invited to the Imperial War Museum. My partner and one of the key members of this group, Ben Helfgott, made the arrangements over the phone for us to meet Ben's sister, Mala, who had been in Belsen. All that I knew was her name and that she had been a child when Belsen was liberated. She had contracted typhus in the 'nursery hut' of the camp and was lucky to survive. She and Ben, who had been in Treblinka, found each other after the war. Their parents and all other family members were killed.

When we got there we looked at the exhibition and as the evening went on I began to realise that I could not possibly find Mala in such a large crowd and with no idea of what she looked like. After the speeches, my partner and I agreed to leave and go home, and as we began to walk towards the exit through the crowded room in which the exhibition was housed, I stopped in front of a woman. As we looked at each other I experienced a strong sense of recognition. 'You're Mala?' I said. 'Yes, and you are Carol', she replied. It always strikes me that I might have imagined that this is how we met, but my partner who witnessed this confirmed that this is the reality.

We talked for a long time and later she told me her story. Mala was keen to meet my father and we arranged for Mala and her husband came to lunch with us and then to drive the 80-odd miles to my parents' house. I wanted some of his wounds to heal and presenting this wonderful, kind and accomplished woman to him was the best way I could find to help. The meeting was special. My father did not speak of Belsen and neither did Mala. As she was leaving the only thing that Mala said to my father about the holocaust was, 'Thank you, for what you did.' He was embarrassed and could not accept that he had done anything at all and dismissed her thanks as unnecessary.

In the last months of my father's life, I went to Belsen on his behalf for a memorial event staged there. I saw for myself the size of the camp, the surrounding woods and tried to imagine what he must have felt and how it could have been possible. I walked into the camp beside a woman who was returning to try to find the grave of her mother who had died two weeks after the liberation, leaving her alone. Although she had great difficulty going back in the camp and froze at the entrance, she eventually found the courage to do so. The camp was enormous and the size of the communal graves beyond imagination. It was also a sterile place, in that there was no evidence of the nightmare of events, except in the museum. Looking at the people who were paying tribute to those who died I saw that they themselves were ageing and recognised the possibility that these living memories would come to an end. I suddenly felt afraid of that loss and realised the importance of not letting the memory of those who died cease to exist.

On the plane home, I sat with a Jewish man who talked about his feelings on seeing Belsen. He had not expected to see a place that was, as he described it, 'sanitised and beautified'. He told me that he expected to see something more horrific, 'like the back of Stanstead airport'. We both laughed at this joke and in that moment I realised the importance of my father's legacy of humour. He made the unmanageable manageable with humour. And that is how I survive the unthinkable and horrific reality of some aspects of life.

71
When Disaster Strikes: Reflections on Personal Experience of Disaster

Disaster Action

This has been written by members of Disaster Action, all of whom are survivors and bereaved people from disasters. Some of the disasters we have been affected by are the Zeebrugge ferry sinking, King's Cross fire, Lockerbie air crash, Hillsborough football stadium crush, Marchioness riverboat sinking, Dunblane shootings, Southall and Ladbroke Grove train crashes, the 11th September attacks, the Tsunami, and the Bali, London 7 July and Sharm El Sheikh bombings.

Some of this may be painful to read, but our intention is to help those who may go through similar reactions after other disasters. We hope it may also help friends and family members to understand the feelings of those they care for. Those who helped us most did not try to 'pigeonhole' us or dictate how we *should* feel.

[...]

Reflections from some survivors

Soon after the event

"The total shock of the event carried us through as did the deeper shock from euphoria at surviving. The 'survivor guilt' you hear about started early and was overwhelming at times. I felt guilt about everything and everyone, but once I could label it as such it started to become easier to deal with. I often wished I had died and reading about funerals and obituaries was like observing my own. A part of me had died and I needed to grieve."

"Obsession with reading every account and watching every video clip of the disaster which comes on the news, etc. Having to record every programme and keep all the newspapers and articles (I have them to this day and they are very precious). I think this is about trying to make it 'real' when the feeling of utter disbelief is so strong and trying to get control back when everything has been out of control and all 'routine' matters of life are gone. Nothing felt normal anymore."

'When Disaster Strikes: Reflections on personal experience of disaster', www.disasteraction.org.uk/support/da_ guide08.pdf, Disaster Action. Reproduced by kind permission of Disaster Action. Survivors and bereaved people from UK and overseas disasters founded Disaster Action (DA) in 1991, as an independent, British-based charity. An advocacy and advisory service, their purpose is to raise awareness of the needs of those directly affected by disaster and to offer support to survivors and bereaved. www.disasteraction.org.uk

After a month or so

"Reports of having a 'glazed' look came up however within a month and the panic attacks and for some people (but not all) flashbacks were so bad as to be crippling and preventing travel, work, or concentration. What was needed was someone to talk to who had been in the accident. Feeling isolated, for some, added to the trauma."

After a few months

"Into the 'recovery' survival, people 'froze' not able to move arms or legs. This was shocking and unexpected in itself. It would have been helpful to have understanding GPs but in some cases they had to learn from us as we went through our journeys."

"We needed information on what the time scales might be to getting some financial support if people had lost jobs or were off work and injuries had led to serious financial hardship."

"Survivors often felt their families and friends had no idea how to deal with these strange people who had returned to live with them. There was no understanding or information available at the time and no support for the families. Survivors also didn't always see that their families were victims of the disaster too, albeit in a different way."

"Collecting belongings was a horrible experience with no understanding of the effect it might have on us. For us there was no information on what would happen and no attempt to single out belongings for individuals was made."

Reflections from some of the bereaved

Soon after the event

"Feeling at times devastated, howling with pain, at times numb with shock, still not quite believing it. Constantly going from one emotion to another, sometimes I am feeling crazy, it is almost a kind of euphoria, like I am free from fear, as the worst thing I could ever have imagined has happened, so now I fear nothing."

"Unable to concentrate on daily routine, I am taking an hour to remember to boil a kettle. I find most foods really hard to contemplate eating, especially meat."

"I am obsessing about how he died. Where was he exactly, did he suffer, did he know he was dying, what was it like for him? Going through it over and over in my mind. Reading every single newspaper every day – they have different stories about how it all happened. I can't work out where he was. I need to find someone who was there, but I daren't ask. Wishing I could have died instead."

"B is coping by working out the statistical probability of him having been there at that time. Tells me it's so close to zero as to be a non-probability. Makes no sense to me, but it is his "mathematical" blokey way of coping."

"Getting his belongings back, everything smelled of soot and ash. Got us closer to him somehow, which sounds really crazy."

"Finding everything I read or watch on TV meaningless. Can't stand soppy sad movies in particular. I went to the library and started reading my way through every book with 'death' in the title. Only things linked with him, it, or death mean anything."

"For the first few months we only wanted to be with people who knew him. Felt angry and impatient with people who are wasting time doing really trivial stuff, like arguing or getting upset with tiny unimportant details. This was not what life was about. We felt such amazing clarity about that."

"Some friends are good and supportive, others run away. I know it must be boring for them to have me wanting to talk about him, and it, all the time. But it's my way of keeping him alive."

"The ongoing trauma seems not to lessen, only change from anger to sadness to numbness and back almost daily."

Some months later

"I found it increasingly hard to relate to anyone who hadn't shared my experience. Friends thought they were doing the right thing by trying to 'make me feel better', which really wasn't helpful. I wanted to talk about my brother's death – where his body was found, who found him and exactly how he had died. My brothers didn't want to talk about these things at all."

"All of us in the family were dealing with it in different ways – the dynamics between us had changed completely."

"People continued to ask me how my parents were, but I felt increasingly – why don't they ask about me? As 'only' a sister, I felt I was pushed down the so-called hierarchy of grief. It did help a bit when people I met from other disasters said the same thing had happened to them."

72

Personal and Medical Memories from Hillsborough

Tom Heller

Outside every public house and on every verge on my way home there were relaxed groups of young men chatting and joking in their 'uniforms' of tight faded jeans, off colour teeshirts, and something red and white. Were these the people whom later I saw laid out on the floor with life just pushed out of them? There were so many I didn't dare count them. They looked as they had in life, not disfigured; they were just lying there, not quite the right colour. Not much to identify them on that sports hall floor. Who were they? What had gone wrong? Who was to blame for all this?

Call for help

I was on call for a practice adjacent to the Hillsborough ground for the weekend of Saturday 15 April. On Saturdays when there is a home match at the stadium I avoid passing the ground when crowds are coming and going. My home is one side of the ground and the practice is on the other. On the 15th the atmosphere was special for the semi-final; people were parking their cars miles away from the stadium and walking to the ground many hours earlier than the crowds usually do for home games. I remember being especially cheerful (despite being on duty) and proud that Sheffield was the centre of the sporting world that day. The snooker world championship was on just down the road, and at Hillsborough the semi-final that many people thought should have been the final of the FA Cup was being held. Both sets of supporters wear red and white; I wonder who was who on those verges and which of them now live to tell their tale of the day when such a terrible tragedy happened out of a relaxed and gentle sunny moment?

I switched on the television just after 3 p.m. and saw the coverage of the snooker being interrupted by scenes from Hillsborough. Like almost everyone else, I imagine, I thought that there had been a pitch invasion and worried about how this might affect the chances of English clubs being allowed back into Europe. I then got into my car and took my daughter to a party that she was due to attend. At about 3.30 p.m. I heard on Radio Sheffield the call for doctors to go to

Tom Heller, 'Personal and medical memories from Hillsborough', in Dickenson, Johnson, Samson Katz (eds), *Death, Dying and Bereavement*, 2nd edn. SAGE, 2000, pp. 371–5. Originally published in BMJ, vol. 299, 1989, pp. 1596–8. Reproduced by permission of *BMJ*.

Hillsborough, so I hurried to drop off my daughter and go to the ground. The party was about 2 km from Hillsborough, and on my way to the ground I followed a fire engine with flashing lights and siren that was going through red traffic lights and on the wrong side of keep left signs. I kept my car glued to the back of the fire engine and was at the ground within a few minutes of hearing the announcement. I parked in Leppings Lane, about 20 m from the blue gate that became such a focus of attention later. I had no notion of the significance of the gate at that time.

As I was parking on the forecourt of a garage that fitted tyres I was approached by some policemen. I told them that there had been a call for doctors on the radio. One of them immediately used his radio to find out where doctors were being asked to go, and we set off, running through the corridors, round the stadium, and towards the sports hall. The stadium was familiar to me as I had often been to matches there. The concrete beneath the grandstands is unusual: it is stained grey, cold and unyielding; the light is always poor beneath the stands, even on sunny afternoons like that one. As we rushed along the atmosphere was all wrong: there were lots of people but there was no noise. We got to the sports hall in about two minutes, and I entered by stepping through a cordon of police officers who were holding back people who were crowding around the outside of the door.

Bodies everywhere

Nothing could have prepared me for the scenes inside. I had thought vaguely that there might be a couple of members of St John Ambulance standing over a man with his head between his knees, telling him to take deep breaths. I had thought that they might have been overwhelmed because four people fainting was more than they could cope with and that I'd join in their exhortations and be back at my daughter's party in time for the second round of the Marmite sandwiches. This was not normal though. There were bodies everywhere. Who was alive and who was dead? They couldn't all be dead. It had to be a mistake: this just didn't happen on sunny afternoons. Blotchy faces against the floor, not disfigured but apparently peaceful. Bodies higgledy-piggledy just inside the door, the line stretching over to the far wall. I asked a policeman what was to be done. Thankfully he pointed away from the bodies to a section of the hall that was separated from them by a long, low screen of the type used to divide sports halls when two different sports are being played at the same time. There were more bodies here though. My God, What could I do? Who was going to tell me what to do?

Without directions I ran along the line of crumpled bodies. At least this lot were alive. I stopped between two bodies, took out my stethoscope, and lifted up a teeshirt and listened, grateful to have the time at last to do something that I knew how to do. I often use 'stethoscope on the chest time' to think during consultations. It's a good ploy really: the patient thinks that I am being ever so thoughtful and thorough, and I have time to think about what the hell to do next. Panic overtook me on this occasion. How could I be sure that this person was the one who needed help most? What was going to happen to all of the others if I stayed with this bloke? I could hear his heartbeat and breath sounds. For some reason I took my stethoscope out my ears and crawled up to his face.

'What's your name, mate?' I asked.

'Terry' was the reply.

'Ok Terry. How are you feeling?'

No answer. Silly question really.

How could I help?

His leg was at the wrong angle somehow, and so was one of his arms; he looked terrible, and where I had rested my stethoscope earlier was obviously not all right at all: it was moving wrongly and was not the right colour either. Although I could hear breath sounds, they were hard to interpret. I think I was just panicking. I remembered how to do a tracheotomy with a Biro. Would this be my opportunity? I turned him over on to his side and pushed my fingers on to the top of his tongue to establish an airway. This seemed to help, and his breathing started again. I had pulled him over on to his bad leg though – there didn't seem much alternative. His face was against the floor, so I reached out and found a leather jacket on the floor and picked up his head and rested it on the jacket. What medical equipment could enable this man to survive? If only someone would arrive who knew what to do. What did I know about anything? I turned around and looked at the man behind me: he was immobile and a terrible blue-grey colour … and so it went on.

I had taken my bags full of the equipment and drugs that I usually use. Not much call for antibiotics or infant paracetamol this afternoon. After some time – how long? – I became aware of a friend of mine going between the bodies doing the same as I was. Another general practitioner. We had worked together in the past but not on anything like this, nor are we likely to again. A smile of recognition. I wonder if I looked as lost as he did.

The first large-scale equipment arrived, and we started working together, putting up drips on everyone. We intubated as many patients and estalished as many airways as we possibly could. We needed scissors to cut through clothes. Why didn't I carry them in my bags? We started giving intravenous diamorphine, and some sort of routine and organization began to be established. I'm quite proud in a funny sort of way to be able to put up so many intravenous drips so quickly without missing a vein. More doctors had arrived by now, and around every body there was a little huddle of workers. Someone said that he was an anaesthetist – gold dust. Come over here and look at Terry for me, mate. He's still alive, but he keeps stopping breathing. 'Hang on, Terry.' The anaesthetist took out the airway, and it was blocked with blood. Not a good sign. One rib seemed to be almost through the chest and was certainly at the wrong angle. The ambulance stretchers arrived, and we put in a passionate bid for Terry to be taken off first. By now six people were around him, holding the drip bottle, his head, and his legs, which were at all angles. He was rested on to a low trolley. I checked that the ambulance was waiting and could get through to the hospital. The anaesthetist went with Terry to the ambulance. Thank God for anaesthetists. I'll never tell an anti-anaesthetist joke again.

Comradeship amid the horror

Now that I had no one to work on I wandered around and could see the dead bodies again at the other side of the sports hall. Among the doctors I recognized many of my friends and colleagues who had also answered the call of duty. One of them gave me a hug, bless him – a friend for life after what we went through that day. The police were much in evidence, but nobody was in charge of the medical tasks. What should I do next? Where would I be most useful? I decided to use my newly refound skills to put up drips on everybody who was going to be transferred to hospital. I somehow remembered that this was the thing to do in case the patients suffered more collapse on the way to hospital. It was also a sign to the hospital doctors that we general practitioners could do something right after all. I used up all of my diamorphine on those in need. By this time the routines were more established. Someone was writing down the obvious major damage to each person and what he or she had received in the way of drugs, etc. Then suddenly there was nobody left in the hall who was in need of attention and who wasn't dead.

I noticed a close friend crouching over amid the sea of dead faces. He was comforting someone who was leaning over a body. I stepped over some bodies to speak to him and offer some help; there weren't any words, just a look of rare empathy and comradeship.

Not knowing how to react

The doctors in the hall grouped together, almost silent, all wondering what to do next. I left the hall and walked through the silent crowds back to my car. I went home stunned and numbed. My children were playing in the garden; it was all so lovely and normal. Sandpits and skipping ropes. I had not known any of the dead or injured. Why is a major disaster so important for the people who participate as helpers? I meet death almost every day of my working life. Was this worse or was it just larger numbers? Everyone sort of expects that an event like this will be upsetting. But why is it that more attention is focused on the feelings of helpers in such disasters than on those of people concerned with upsetting events that happen every day? For me it seems to have been a major shock to my system in a general sort of way. I was grumpy, washed out and flat for a couple of weeks. Passing Hillsborough shocked me again for a long while afterwards when I had nearly rebuilt my professional defences.

All of us general practitioners who were there met a few times to talk about our experiences and to support each other. Why are all the others so articulate about how they are feeling whereas I'm just sort of non-specifically upset? I can't remember what I felt like at the ground and can't describe to the helpful counsellor how I'm feeling during the group sessions. I know all the theory, but I can't get it together for myself – the plight of the modern professional. It's three weeks since the disaster now, and I'm feeling OK again; I make jokes at work and have lots to be thankful for. I've been enormously well supported through all this by family, friends and colleagues. Time has passed and lessons to be learnt are being thought about. Perhaps British football has changed because of these events, and perhaps major disasters will be better dealt with in the future.

I'd like to tell the official inquiry in a systematic way what I think went right with the medical response that day and what I think could be done better next time. I don't know what training should be given to general practitioners and why none of us took charge of the medical happenings in the sports hall and was prepared to be the coordinator. I've got strong views about the counselling that is necessary and appropriate after the event for helpers at disasters. I'd like to do physical damage to the person who took the pictures for the *Daily Mirror* and reserve a special act of aggression for the person who allowed them to be published. But most of all I'd like to find out what happened to Terry.

73
The Personal and Professional Reflections of a Forensic Ecologist

Patricia Wiltshire

Other than the demise of my brother's goldfish, my first awareness of death was at the age of ten when my father's relatively young parents followed each other in rapid succession. I was surprised at my parents' tears since I only felt vague sorrow. Each grandparent had a traditional, Welsh, black funeral, with drawn curtains in every house in the street, masses of flowers, and genuine, respectful sadness from neighbours. I was impressed by the solemnity and theatre of the proceedings, but certainly enjoyed the ensuing get-together of family and friends. The contrast of sadness and jollity left me somewhat bemused.

True bereavement first hit me years later when my maternal grandmother was killed in an accident; my strict, clever, practical, capable, warm, loving, generous grandmother. I was grown up, but remember the acute shock of realising, even so, she would no longer be there to protect me from the ills of the world. I felt that I now had to take emotional responsibility for myself and others. Even though it may have been irrational, for the first time I felt alone and frightened. I had never even contemplated that she might, one day, leave me: the suddenness of her departure was unreal. I wasn't even able to attend her funeral because my nine-month old daughter had become ill; that illness was the precursor of the shaping of my whole attitude, not only to death, but to 'the world, universe, and everything'. A rare, malignant disease took her away from me ten months later; ten months of intense pain and suffering for her and for us, her doting parents.

My daughter's death was another unreal event, and so close to the first. Gentle nurses roused me and took me to her. She wasn't dead! I could see her breathing! I sat there staring in numbed disbelief until the same gentle nurses led me away to another room. No, she was *not* breathing – and never would again. My beautiful, blond, rosy-cheeked child had truly left me for ever. I felt an electric shock and then the draining away of my insides. Not everything that left me ever came back. There is still an overwhelming void that nothing will fill or satisfy. The worse thing that could ever happen to me had happened. No disaster or misfortune would ever have the same impact, or ever hurt me as much.

I cannot dwell on the loss of my child; it is too painful. But it certainly had a potent impact on my whole attitude to life and death. No one else's parting would ever affect me as intensely or in the same way. No one and nothing could ever hurt me as much, and this meant that, in a strange way, I was protected from future ills.

As one gets older, one collects bereavements, and the passing of other family members each played a role in my perception of the dying process, and of death itself.

I found my father-in-law's dying a very interesting experience. I was fond of him and, as his end approached, I tried to lift him into a more comfortable position. I found his fluttering pulse and was interested by the irregularity of its rhythm and strength. The last rapid quivers coincided with his giving a single gasp and staring me full in the face. With this last breath all animation left him. I was fascinated by the change. He was Dad – and then just a body; this happened within a blink. I had the same experience with my mother-in-law many years later. As she was dying, she was very much a person, but she became an 'it' within seconds. In both cases, the contrast was stark. But it was quite comforting to me to realise that the dead body is simply an empty vessel; a bottle from which all the spirit has drained. My own mother's death simply reinforced my view, and I was doubly comforted to know that she thought the same as me. It surprised me that I could regard the deaths of those of whom I was fond with such dispassion and objectivity. But then, I was shielded by my former, excruciatingly painful experiences. All of them helped to form my attitude to the human body.

At one level, I feel that only a body with life has meaning; a dead one is for recycling, and it is easy and convenient to think like this when one is dealing with death on a regular basis and in a professional capacity. But, I have to admit that when I think of the two people who have meant most to me, my daughter and maternal grandmother, there is a chink in this armour of detachment. In spite of my clinical objectivity, their deaths make it obvious to me that one must respect the feelings of all those who have lost loved ones, irrespective of the way they were lost.

I needed to fill the void left by the death of my daughter and decided to go to university. I had a wonderful training as an ecologist at King's College London where my passion and curiosity for the natural world were indulged and facilitated by the dedicated experts there. I was given the opportunity to study any aspect of any biological and ecological subject on offer, and for years I was immersed in academia – far removed from the harsh reality of having to apply my knowledge to make a living. I eventually became a lecturer at King's College and, looking back, I think that being an academic was (and is) such a luxury and privilege. After my experiences of the last 14 years, I realise that it was a very easy existence.

Applying science has always interested me more than science for its own sake, and I eventually moved to the Institute of Archaeology, in University College London, where I was engaged in reconstructing past environments by microscopical analysis of archaeological deposits. This offered new challenges and many excitements. As a botanical ecologist and palynologist (pollen analyst), I was able to create pictures of past landscapes, farming practices, and the domestic status of ancient peoples. It was heady and exciting, especially as I was invited to participate in excavations of wonderful sites ranging from the Palaeolithic (Old Stone Age) to historical times. From my analytical data, I was able to provide mental images of the pre-Roman and Roman landscape and economies at Hadrian's Wall, Pompeii, Godmanchester, Druidic sites in Colchester, and many others. I could actually 'see' the past from assemblages of pollen grains and spores extracted from soil, mud, muck, vessels and bones. These microscopic particles were derived from the plants growing at the same time that ancient people were living, so by being able to build up information on past vegetation, I was able to reconstruct the nature of the archaeological environment. By relentless hard work, and being able to envisage the past from looking at sheets of numbers derived from microscopical analysis, I was pre-adapted for a most unexpected twist of fate and change of direction.

One day, I received a telephone call from a police officer who asked me if I could tell him whether or not a car had driven into a field where the burnt remains of a corpse had been found in a ditch. I was fascinated. I didn't know whether I could help or not, but I would certainly try. To everyone's surprise (my own included), not only could I tell that the occupants of the car *had* been into that field, but could also pin-point the precise area of ditch from which they had picked up the tiny amounts of soil I had found from the vehicle. My work provided the police with sufficient intelligence to be able to challenge a gang of drug dealers, and further enquiries led to their conviction. This case gave birth to the disciplines of 'environmental profiling' and 'forensic palynology' which I have been developing and refining ever since.

I have now been involved with around 200 criminal cases and have worked with most of the police forces in the whole of the United Kingdom. Previously, I had attempted to fill my void by the vicarious excitements offered by archaeology. Although 'excitement' is not a wholly appropriate word, I was soon to find that murder, rape, abduction and searching for graves and human remains would replace archaeology in filling my attention.

Quite frankly, some of the investigations have provided me a great deal of 'academic fun' – an ecological equivalent of Sudoko. But while obtaining and interpreting analytical results provide perversely enjoyable intellectual challenges, everything else associated with such investigations is difficult and stressful, both physically and mentally.

For me, a murder might start with a telephone call at the crack of dawn to attend a scene where the mangled, rotting body of a girl had been found by a dog-walker the night before. Trampling or disturbance will destroy important environmental evidence that might have otherwise been available, but those police investigators who are aware of what forensic ecology can offer will wait until I can get there.

But what of my personal reaction to the numerous murders and corpses I encounter?

I consider myself to be a normal woman, but with an exceptionally robust approach to people, life and death. On many occasions I have been required to do things, and be involved with situations, that have made even tough police officers cringe.

I frequently deal with corpses of people who have suffered violent attack; they may be dismembered or mutilated. Whether one is helping to excavate human remains, or lift a corpse out of leaf litter, or getting trace evidence from the body in the harsh, clinical light of the mortuary, the experience never fails to be strangely unreal. It requires a particular mental approach – and a strong stomach.

In nearly every case, I am detached from the possibility that the body lying in front of me might have been a real person. I see it as an empty vessel, just as I did with my parents-in-law and my own mother. I cannot afford to allow myself to think of these poor unfortunates as anything other than 'an investigation'. To a large extent, I am protected from experiences that would be frightening and sickening to most. I see my contribution as a useful cog in the wheels of the investigation. But, there have been exceptions.

Of all the cadavers I have seen in the course of my work, three live with me; they touched me to the point of tears. One was a beautiful, innocent, young Scandinavian girl, a victim of the frantic lust of a man she had had the misfortune to meet as she was picking wild flowers. She was 'a sleeping beauty' as she lay in the mortuary. The other was a prostitute; she had never had any security or loving comfort in her short life. She was emaciated, dirty, and hopelessly addicted to cocaine. The reason for her prostitution was drugs, but also that she was trying to maintain her three young children, and protect them from her pimp. The third was a six-month-old bonny baby boy who had had a feckless mother and resentful stepfather. Although I have worked on the corpses of many children, the post-mortem of this child disturbed me deeply for a long time.

I have come to realise that my feelings about the bodies of victims of crime depends partly on the state of the body. I certainly find it easier to cope with decomposed corpses and dismembered body parts than fresh, whole bodies. If the victim looks merely asleep, it is much harder than if the corpse is in pieces, or has started to decompose. I suppose if the body has already started to become detritus, the human is difficult to identify. The other potent factor in the impact the body has on me is the relative innocence of the victim. Many of those having suffered violent death are known, in life, to have been as vicious and threatening as those who killed them. The true innocents just do not deserve to have their lives taken from them prematurely by anyone. I feel this very strongly, and my own deep bereavements must be affecting my attitudes here.

It would seem that I have variable resilience. As a consequence, I do suffer. But someone has to do the job …

74

Returning Property After Death and Disaster

Lucy Easthope

The return of personal property after death and disaster is all about *things*; things that are important to people, that represent the last link to their loved one. These items are not necessarily of any financial value, and it's important to remember that this process is not about money or recompense or insurance (although insurers will sometimes help to pay for the process.) It might be a T-shirt, a pair of jeans, a cheap watch, one earring, a credit card, a teddy bear, a receipt or, very occasionally, a love letter.

Items of this nature are returned every day; Police Family Liaison Officers, staff at hospitals and hospices and Coroner's Officers will all be involved with returning property after death. It might be a sudden death in a road traffic accident or after many months of an illness. Disasters tend to magnify the issues because of the amount of property and the higher likelihood of damage to the items. It is also more difficult to remember that each family is individual when there are hundreds, and even thousands, of families for the responders to correspond with.

I will never forget the first time that I collected the property retrieved from the wreckage of a disaster in the United Kingdom. All those who had died were men, and their property represented some sort of generalisation of their age, their gender; racy magazines, big canvas bags, branded underpants. I have worked with grieving families, in the mortuary, as the administrator repatriating remains from overseas. My colleagues warned me that of all of these things the 'hardest' work would be the process of returning personal effects, and I think they may have been right. It felt like a huge invasion of privacy, not just of one person, but of a whole family. And it was very close to home. Collecting me from the warehouse, every evening, was my husband, of near identical age to those men who had died, with a wash bag that mirrored the ones before me – the razor blades, the Gillette shaving foam, the Colgate, the way that the bottom of a bag probably bought by mum or grandad several years earlier had gathered a thin layer of soap and fluff. It was those bags that I remember the most.

Do people even know that this sort of work goes on? That in several locations around the country there are storage facilities packed with the belongings of those who have been involved in a tragedy. Working in disaster management you learn to accept that your sense of normality and reason will be challenged, that you will see things that don't make sense at first glance. Nothing can prepare you for walking into a room where bank notes are drying on a washing line (after crashes, explosions and other similar events, a lot of the property may be wet and foamy due to the fire fighting methods) and on every table there are trays of keys and shoes and wallets and hairbrushes and buttons that just days ago were such a small part of someone's life but now might represent the only thing that you can give back to a grieving parent, partner, child or friend. That's another thing about this work; the human body is a fragile thing and may be almost completely destroyed in a fire, but a passport or a piece of jewellery could survive almost completely intact.

One of my most memorable 'returns' was being given a pile of wet clothing that revealed a tiny scrap of paper. There were no obvious markings on it but I put it on some gauze to dry and as it did so, slowly peeled it open. It was a very personal letter from a man to his wife. I dried it out with a hair dryer on the lowest setting. I noticed that it was signed off with a pet name similar to one that I used for my own husband, that I have been unable to use since. It was returned to the wife and usually I would hear no more after that point, but about a week later I saw the widow on the local news holding up the letter and saying that it had been a great comfort to know that he had it with him when he died.

It is not simply a case of gathering up the property and returning it. Many police forces continue to 'censor' the property that they recover after any death. They apply their own sensibilities to the item, for example: 'I would not want it back with blood stains on it so neither will the mother' (who until a week ago they had never met before). These judgement calls also mean that they remove condoms or Viagra from the inventory because they are 'rude and embarrassing'. I am regularly challenged on this aspect of my work and I don't always have the answers. I have consulted with senior military personnel who maintain that they will always remove pornography, letters that could cause distress (for example, to a boyfriend when there is also a wife) and anything else that they consider inappropriate. Illegality also causes problems; guns, fake passports, cocaine found within a suitcase belonging to a deceased person – but usually the process allows for sensitive handling. Counterfeiting can also be a problem if you attempt to return an item, such as a fake watch, to the maker for repair, believing it to be real, and they destroy it on principle.

In the past, items have been destroyed without consultation, or laundered with plenty of flowery smelling conditioner to ensure that there is no trace of the smell of burning or body fluids. It is about choice. Some families may prefer the latter but, for others, the last connection to their loved one is irreversibly taken away. If families are asked first, then they can decide. It is easier to make a blanket decision and blame it on 'health and safety' and 'evidential reasons'. Recent good practice after disasters in the UK illustrate that both of these can often be overcome. A good responder will always check first. Responders such as Police Family Liaison Officers can talk to the families about the items and show them photographs and, with the right legal guidance, a future court case does not need to be compromised by returning the property, and effects do not need to be stored indefinitely.

It is daunting to design a process that will ensure an individualised approach to 30,000 items. (To reach an approximate number of items, list separately everything you are wearing, then add to that everything in your wallet and remember each item is managed separately, every bank card, 5 pence piece, lipstick, then do the same for your handbag or briefcase and your suitcase.) Forms and protocols have to be designed and administered, and if families do want items to be laundered, cleaned, or repaired, then that has to be facilitated. There should always be the option to have items returned 'as is' or as close to that as possible (our approach to death seems very sanitised in the western world, but undertakers have always been a very useful source of advice and support to me; with their help, items can still be returned safely as close to their original condition as possible).

There can be a jarring clash between sensitivity and operational requirement (mirroring other aspects of the process after sudden death, such as evidence gathering and court procedure). Forms need to be signed and legal 'next of kin ' needs to be determined. The most clinical part of the process comes near the end when there are thousands of items with no obvious owner. A catalogue is produced and these days we use technology like laptops and CD-Roms, but I still cannot imagine what it must be like to sit and view that, looking out for something you might recognise. Then you have to make a claim on that item and if there are 'multiple claims' on that one item, a panel of lawyers and insurers may be convened to adjudicate. Once, there were 19 claims for a biro with a chewed end. It was heart-breaking to think that all around the world (this was an air crash involving numerous nationalities) there were people thinking 'I remember him/her with that pen, just chewing on it as they thought'.

Items have previously been returned in bin bags and evidence bags. The Metropolitan Police are leading on a project to ensure that items are returned in a more sensitive and appropriate way, using beautiful boxes, and there are other examples of best practice all around the country. This happens every day. Then you have to decide how long you will store unclaimed property for, or property that the families simply are not ready to look at.

It would be wrong to imply that this is an organised, assumed process that automatically happens after every disaster in the UK. In the USA they have the Aviation Disaster Family Assistance Act 1996 which safeguards people's right to have property returned after air disasters, but in the UK, we only have guidance.

The return of personal property owes much to dedicated individuals, who educate themselves about the requirements after disaster, and ensure that the process happens. Sometimes they have to fight authority to get it going. In my work I occasionally encounter opposition to it, although people are becoming much more aware now. There are numerous articles expounding the importance of a rights-based approach for bereaved families, the protection of their right to choose. We have come a long way, but I still see plans and planners that are imbued with an alarming amount of 'paternalism'. It is not about what you and I want. It is an individual's choice.

Lucy Easthope is a Disaster Management Consultant and has worked for several employers including the Metropolitan Police.

75
Collective Loss and Community Resilience After September 11

Anne Eyre

'Mind-blowing' ... 'searing emotional pain' ... 'aftershock'. These are some of the ways in which the attacks on the World Trade Centre in New York on September 11 2001 and their immediate aftermath have been described. In New York City alone 2,973 lives were lost, with countless more people impacted (Greene et al., 2006: 1).

So what was the impact of such sudden and unexpected mass death on those directly affected through such traumatic bereavement? How did the City and surrounding areas respond from such a catastrophic event in the longer term, and what can we learn for dealing with the effects of mass fatalities in future? These were among the questions explored through my Churchill Fellowship Travels to New York and New Jersey in June/July 2006. Almost five years after the event I met representatives from the New York police and fire departments, emergency management departments, the British Consulate, and the American Red Cross, as well as university researchers, to learn about the impacts of mass traumatic loss from that day onwards.

The experiential journey I made during my visit was a deeply personal voyage as well as a professional one. A retired fire-fighter who, like most people I met, had both personal and professional links to the disaster on 9/11, showed me around Ground Zero and took me to see the new fire-fighters' memorial there. It was particularly poignant to learn about that day and its aftermath from those with direct personal experience, and on that occasion to be shown the site by someone who had been in the towers many times as a professional fire-fighter. No one I met during my meetings was unaffected by this work, though all demonstrated remarkable resilience in the face of adversity. This emerges as a key theme in the recovery of those involved in disasters.

Understanding the context of mass death

It was interesting to me to find that Israel's response to terrorist events was frequently referred to by my American colleagues. Much advice was made available by Israeli consultants after 9/11, and this proved most helpful given their historical experience of ongoing terrorism. In particular we discussed the contrasting approach to disaster sites, which reflects both the political and social meaning attached to events and their location. In Israel, the site of a bombing is deliberately cleaned up and 'normalised' within hours; at locations such as Ground Zero and other commemorative sites in the US and UK, such sites become memorialised and the focus for political and cultural debates about the nature and significance of continued remembrance and commemoration.

My discussions reinforced the importance placed in our Western cultures of symbolically marking sites and giving families affected by events choices and control in relation to personal and public ritual and remembrance. We also discussed how commemoration can have negative effects for individuals, for example, schoolchildren who lost parents at the World Trade Centre may feel singled out for attention every year when classroom silences are observed and banners everywhere remark on the need to 'Never Forget 9/11'.

Discussing the fifth anniversary of 9/11 and the controversies that continue in relation to the long-term plans for the site, I was struck by the contrast between this and Israel's approach, both of which testify in different ways to the cultural meaning attached to the marking of events. Being in New York on the first anniversary of the July 7 bombings in London and away from home was also a poignant point of reflection for me.

Personal testimony and interventions

I feel privileged to have been able to listen to first-hand personal accounts of what happened in the first few minutes, hours and days on 9/11. These were shared by those who had seen the collapse of the twin towers with their own eyes and became part of the response and recovery effort over the weeks, months and years that followed.

Much of disaster mental health focuses disproportionately on extreme negative reactions following such direct experiences, but these accounts highlighted for me how resilient people can be in the face of collective death and dying. Those I met described the many tasks they and their colleagues undertook, often spontaneously and with little explicit professional planning and training, for example, triaging medical and psychological emergencies, evacuating victims from the immediate vicinity of Ground Zero, staffing help-lines, coordinating family assistance centres, and distributing food and other supplies to the uniformed service workers who were searching for survivors from the first few days onwards. Their reflections and details of the scale and logistics associated with responding to the disaster highlighted the unique scale and impact of these events.

The effects of September 11

'You could have known 100 people who died that day; some people don't even know 100 people ...' This comment made by one of New York's fire-fighters and peer counsellors during one of my meetings illustrates the very extensive impact of the events on September 11 on those in New York and New Jersey. The ripple effects extend well beyond the immediate geographical area of the financial district of Manhattan. One quarter of all the victims lost in the World Trade Centre were residents of New Jersey. Thus 'September 11 is a New Jersey story as much as a New York, Washington, or Pennsylvania story. For the families of the 691 residents killed on 9/11, there is no distinction, no state line' (Crimando and Padro, 2005: 107). As well as the extensive loss of life and traumatic impacts on survivors, the extensive economic impacts, political consequences and other ripple effects were huge.

The City's Fire Department (FDNY) lost 343 of it members, representing the largest loss of life of any emergency response agency in history. Many of those who survived remained actively involved in the nine-month body recovery mission, a harrowing duty but one dictated by their strong culture and tradition by which they have always recovered their own. 'To take away their mission would have been to deprive them of purpose at a time when they were suffering tremendous trauma and loss ... Finding a recovery gave them both a sense of accomplishment and a horrific memory' (Greene et al., 2006: 65).

As with the UK, members of the emergency services have traditionally been hostile to 'mental health' professionals from outside of their own community addressing them in the aftermath of incidents. Within the emergency response community in New York, the principles of peer-based strategies were adopted as a key element in community-based approaches to psycho-social support. As with the outreach to families, this was a bereavement situation like no other. Some of the most difficult aspects of this disaster included traumatic elements: the long search for remains, the loss of family members and multiple friends, continuing intrusive reminders by the media and others, and the public scrutiny of private grief (Greene et al., 2006: 181). The loss of fire-fighter fathers such as 'Mr Mom' – who had actively co-parented during their days off – threatened to further destabilise families losing a primary caregiver (Greene et al., 2006: 187).

Recognising that prolonged and intense exposure might have long term after-effects, New York's Police Department (NYPD) offered its officers the opportunity of physical and psychological health checks after the Ground Zero recovery operation closed in June 2002. Like so many of the support strategies I heard about, the procedures involved here were innovative, necessitated by the unique nature and context of the work these officers were undertaking. The Director of the Psychological Evaluation Unit was impressed by how hardy and resilient the officers were shown to be; he commented on their *esprit de corps* and how the exaggerated reports of post-traumatic stress disorder can often distort the real picture. 'I think resilience is under-rated' he said, and we went on to discuss the growing literature and evidence of resilience and post-traumatic growth in studies of disaster responders. Our discussion highlighted that support for those who undertook the recovery work, who were designated as 'heroes', was clearly one of the factors which enhanced the coping skills of those undertaking this task.

The Port Authority of New York and New Jersey lost 37 of its police officers and 47 of their civilian staff, who all died on 9/11. I met senior officers from its Medical Services who shared their personal and professional experiences of the day. Both had also been with the organisation during the attack on the World Trade Centre on February 26, 1993. I was impressed not only by their personal testimonies but also the sensitivity incorporated in the support services offered to bereaved families of their employees. These included the establishment of family assistance centres at airports, the deployment of a family liaison officer to each of the victims' families, staff debriefings and community-based support groups. They also shared their experiences of dealing with the media after they were forced to release transcripts of emergency calls made on the morning of 9/11. Events like these were among the most traumatic for families, and explain why the years after the attacks have had such continuing effects on staff.

One of my colleagues who responded after 9/11 commented on the resonance then of the following quote from Churchill. It emphasises preparing for the chance to turn future mass tragedies into opportunities and to make a positive difference:

> To every [man] there comes in [his] lifetime that special moment when [he is] figuratively tapped on the shoulder and offered [a] chance to do a very special thing, unique to [him] and [fitted to his] talents. What a tragedy if that moment finds [him] unprepared or unqualified for [that] which [would be his] finest hour. (Sir Winston Churchill)

References

Crimando, S. and Padro, G. (2005) 'Across the River: New Jersey's Response to 9/11' in Y. Danieli (ed.) (2005) *On the Ground after September 11: Mental Health Responses and Practical Knowledge Gained.* New York: Haworth Press.

Eyre, A. (2006) *Community Support after Disasters.* Report of a Winston Churchill Travelling Fellowship to the United States of America. Available at www.wcmt.org.uk/public/reports/ 60_1.pdf.

Greene, P., Kane, D., Christ, G., Lynch, S. and Corrigan, M. (2006) *FDNY Crisis Counselling: Innovative Responses to 9/11 Firefighters, Famlies and Communities.* Hoboken, NJ: Wiley.

Part VII

Making Sense of the After-Life and Life After Death

Introduction

Sarah Earle and Carol Komaromy

Across different times, places and cultures people have expressed a strong need to understand what lies beyond death. Is death simply 'the end' or does some part of us live on in another world? Can those who die communicate with the living? Are the dead reborn? All of these questions – and many others – are subject to continuous debate and are central to religious and spiritual ideologies. Some faiths offer certainty about life after death and the form that it will take. Other faiths have documented the route or journey to the next life. Most belief systems offer guidance on how to behave in order to achieve immortality. These questions can be important to those who are dying (and living), as well as to those who care for them. They are also relevant in the immediate aftermath of a death and in the time beyond. Part VII offers examples of the ways in which people make sense of the after-life and life after death.

Many people will have personal experience – or will know someone with personal experience – of apparitions. There are many different types of apparition, but the first piece in this Part is drawn from a database which documents paranormal activity (www.paranormaldatabase.com). The database has 7,700 entries of paranormal activity; the extracts presented here are from the section on 'hospital ghosts and hauntings', which are very commonly reported types of apparition. While in western societies many are sceptical, the concept of apparitions has a long history; for example, they are mentioned in the books of the Old and New Testaments. Apparitions also continue to capture the popular imagination in films such as *Poltergeist*, *Ghost* and *Casper* and in the *Harry*

Potter books and films by J.K. Rowling. In the next piece, which has been specially commissioned for this volume, Suzanne Perry tells the story of her family's ghosts. Whilst she does not doubt that her family members experienced what they claimed, she offers another explanation for these ghostly sightings. Turning next to the subject of deathbed apparitions, in a newly commissioned piece, Simon J. Sherwood argues that while such experiences have been collected for over a century, little is actually known about why such experiences occur – although he offers several possible explanations. The next piece, an extract from the book *The Traveller-Gypsies* by Judith Okely, discusses the role of the 'mulo' (ghost or dead person) in the mortuary rites of Travellers, exploring this in the context of identity and social organisation within their culture.

For some people, communicating or connecting with someone who has died is important, and the following two pieces explore this issue. The first piece is an edited extract from the book *If the Spirit Moves You* by Justine Picardie. Here the author describes some of her many attempts to contact her dead sister Ruth and the urgency of this task. In the second piece to focus on this issue, which has been newly commissioned, Jo Dawson asks the question: 'Is anybody there?' and tells her family's story of visiting a spiritualist.

Not everybody believes in an after-life or seeks to make sense of it, but life after death must be faced by all those who lose someone close to them. In the next piece, mother and daughter – Dorothy Thornton and Gayle Letherby – write about the death of Ron, husband and father, and the long life they have built following his death. Of course, when someone dies, many people seek to commemorate and memorialise the life of that person. In the piece 'Sparkling epitaphs', journalist Roger Dobson explores diamonds, fireworks and some of the other contemporary ways of celebrating someone's life (see also the images in Part I; Anna Davidsson Brembourg in Part II; and Anne Eyre in Part VI).

76
Hospital Ghosts and Hauntings

Paranormal Database

Sally
Location: Barnsley (Yorkshire) – Barnsley District Hospital
Type: Haunting Manifestation
Date/Time: Unknown
Further Comments: Said to be built on the site of a poorhouse, the sounds of children wailing can be heard on the Infections Disease ward. A ghost nicknamed Sally haunts another area of the hospital and reportedly touches the side of anyone who enters the side room in which she died, while an area of offices is home to a friendly phantom old lady who sits in a rocking chair.

Grey Figure
Location: Birmingham (West Midlands) – Birmingham & Midland Eye Centre, City Hospital
Type: Haunting Manifestation
Date/Time: 1996
Further Comments: During the building's construction, CCTV picked up the image of a strange grey figure – security was sent to the scene, but no one could be found. A ward sister was encountered along a top floor corridor only visible from the knees upwards. Around the same time, a crew of workers found themselves locked in a room after investigating cries heard from within; once again nothing could be found. A priest was finally summoned to the area.

Drug Induced Ghost
Location: Cambridge (Cambridgeshire) – Addenbrookes Hospital
Type: Haunting Manifestation
Date/Time: Unknown
Further Comments: The story is that a ghost appears to those who are being administrated morphine; the psychological effects of the drug would appear to be ignored in this tale …

Footsteps
Location: Chorley (Lancashire) – Chorley Hospital
Type: Crisis Manifestation
Date/Time: November 1968
Further Comments: Phantom footsteps and the sounds of doors opening and slamming brought staff running in the maternity wing, just in time to discover and save a baby from suffocation.

Victorian Nurse
Location: Exeter (Devon) – Hospital
Type: Haunting Manifestation
Date/Time: Unknown
Further Comments: A ghostly nurse occasionally appears by the bed of anyone close to death and rearranges any nearby flowers so that they form a cross.

Excerpts from 'Hospital ghosts and hauntings', Paranormal Database (www.paranormaldatabase.com/reports/hospital.php). Reproduced by kind permission of Darren Mann.

77
Family Ghosts

Suzanne Perry

Within my extended family there are several ghost stories. The first one of interest is that of my Aunt Sarah. Twenty-one years ago my maternal great-grandfather, Abuelo Antonio, had been ill for some time and died just before my Aunt Sarah's 14th birthday. Sarah's mum (my maternal grandmother and Abuelo's daughter) travelled to Spain to be with him in hospital before he died. Abuelo Antonio was very keen for Sarah to visit him as they had been close, however, Sarah's mum wouldn't allow her the time off school and sadly, he passed away. Sarah was 'very upset' that she 'didn't get to see him before he died' as he had wanted, and although it wasn't her fault, said she felt guilty.

The following summer, Aunt Sarah travelled to Spain with her family, as they did every year, and stayed in Abuelo's house. One night she went to bed quite early; her sister Alison (my mother), with whom she always shared a room, was out with friends. As Aunt Sarah lay in bed, Abuelo 'suddenly appeared' before her. She felt frightened and quickly hid under the sheet. She told me she asked herself: 'Why should I be frightened, it's only Abuelo, I needn't be scared'. And so (quite bravely) she 'peeped over the covers, where he was still hovering and smiling by the foot of her bed'. She remembers him not being solid but appearing ghostly and in a shimmering light, and after what must have been only a few seconds, he disappeared. She knows now that he had come to say goodbye and to let her know that he was 'pleased that she had returned to see him'. My aunt's guilt about not seeing Abuelo before he died reduced after her encounter with his ghost.

Some years later, in 2003, my sister Maria was eight when Grandmamma Flo, our paternal great-grandmother, died. It was the first death in the family that she had been old enough to understand and it affected her as much as you might expect – lots of tears and general ill-ease. Contemplating the after-life and coming to terms with the complete loss of someone who'd been there their whole life is an emotional experience for anyone, let alone an 8-year-old! Months after Grandmamma Flo's death, Maria was brushing her hair when she felt 'something' behind her. As she looked into the mirror, behind her right shoulder she briefly saw Grandmamma Flo's face. Like my Aunt Sarah, Maria recalls my great-grandmother smiling. She wasn't scared, rather she felt her presence to be a comfort of sorts; Maria told me that seeing the image of our late great-grandmother smiling proved to her that she was 'happy' and that Maria was 'not to worry'.

I can't help but wonder that perhaps these sightings were the manifestations of young grieving minds overloaded with uncertainty and guilty feelings? But what about the older and more mature members of my family? They too have had visits from the deceased – but what does this mean to them?

My Nan (on my mother's side) has always been a Catholic and a highly spiritual person. She has controversially experimented with Ouija boards, can read tarot cards and has had premonitions of minor events in her dreams. Her belief in the after-life is very strong; for example, she recalls one night many years ago, as she was drifting off to sleep, that my Grandfather's recently deceased Aunt – Tita Emilia – called out to her, asking for help. She managed to sleep that night but ran to the nearest church early the next morning to light a candle to help Tita Emilia's soul rest in peace.

Most prominent for her, though, was the encounter she had with her late mother (my maternal grandmother). In 2004, my Nan's mother, Luisa, had been fighting breast cancer with many operations for nearly 15 years, and my Nan had been caring for her at home throughout. Abuela Luisa would frequently say how scared she was of dying and although my family did all they could to comfort her, it did little to calm her angst. It was extremely important for my Nan that she was with her mother when she died, but sadly Luisa's last few hours were unpleasant and deeply traumatic and she died in an ambulance on the way to the hospital. My Nan was deeply distressed that her scared, dying mother hadn't been in her arms at the moment of death, and the guilt she felt was strong.

A number of months after Luisa's death, my Nan was restlessly lying in bed when she felt a 'heavy body' lying in bed next to her; she felt the presence of her mother. My Nan then heard Luisa let out a small restful sigh and ever since then she was reassured that her mother was no longer in pain and was 'rested', wherever she might be.

The strangest of family ghost stories are the ones told by those you wouldn't expect. For example, when I listened to my (paternal) Grandad Joe, straight-laced, set in his ways and forever the sceptic when it comes to things of this nature, talk about his own ghostly encounter with a late aunt of my Nan – Tita Maria – the sceptic in me vanished and my spiritual self felt the hairs on the back of my neck stand on end.

My Nan's family owns the open air cinema in the Spanish town they live in, La Linea, and several generations of the family have lived in the house attached to the cinema. My Nan and Grandad now own the house and let it to tenants. Last year, Grandad Joe was at the house doing some repairs when he heard what he thought was the tenant say something he couldn't quite make out. He turned and saw a figure crossing the corridor going out of the house. He asked the figure he assumed was the new tenant, 'Where are you going?' The figure looked like my Nan's aunt, Tita Maria, who had lived her entire life in the house on the other side of the cinema. She turned to my granddad and simply said 'No! I'm sorting out my drawers', and then disappeared.

My Grandad's story stands aside from that of my aunt's, sister's and Nan's; there was no 'need' for Tita Maria to appear to my Grandad, in that it didn't alleviate guilt, ease a naïve troubled soul or put him at much needed rest as it had done for them.

I take an open minded view of these sightings. I've taken heed to the principles of testament and never doubted that my family members had experienced what they claimed. I've been critical in that I've pondered the possibility of these 'ghosts' being products of adventurously imaginative and over-loaded young/grieving minds. However, I believe that my Grandad's story stands as relative proof; he had no connection to Tita Maria's death, no pending unresolved inner feelings. Perhaps, then, there actually are such things as ghosts? At least ... there is in my family!

78
Deathbed Apparitions

Simon J. Sherwood

Shortly before they die, some people on their deathbeds report seeing apparitions of deceased relatives and friends, unknown people or religious figures. In some instances, visions of environmental scenes, often interpreted as images of an after-life, are described. Music or singing can sometimes be reported too. Examples of such deathbed experiences have been collected indirectly via family members and medical personnel for over a century (e.g. Barrett, 1926/1986; Bozzano, 1906; Brayne et al., 2006; Ethier, 2005; Giovetti, 1982; Hyslop, 1908; Morse with Perry, 1994; Myers, 1889; Osis, 1961; Osis and Haraldsson, 1986; Snell, 1928; Turner, 1959). In some cases, these experiences are also witnessed by those present at the bedside (e.g. Barrett, 1926/1986: Chapter III; Bozzano, 1906: 84; Morse with Perry, 1994: 69–70; Myers, 1889; Snell, 1928: 33–9, 59–63); rarer still are cases in which those present report seeing a cloudy substance or 'astral body' leave the patient's body at the point of death (see Barrett, 1926/1986: Chapter VI). Of particular interest are cases in which the dying person reports seeing an apparition of a person they did not know was actually dead (e.g. Bozzano, 1906: 78; Hyslop, 1908: 88–9; Morse with Perry, 1994: 25). These deathbed apparitions typically communicate to the dying person that they have come to collect them and help them cross over to the next stage of their existence (see Hyslop, 1908: 83; Osis and Haraldsson, 1986: 84). Generally, the resulting emotions experienced by the dying person during these encounters are very positive – including feelings of peace, happiness, excitement and a lack of fear of dying – and they are happy to go along with their visitors' wishes. However, in some cases individuals are frightened and don't wish to go with them (e.g., Ethier, 2005; Osis and Haraldsson, 1986). Sometimes dying people reach out toward the apparition; this can be one of their last actions before they die (see Ethier, 2005: 108).

These deathbed experiences can be intensely spiritual experiences that have a considerable impact upon the dying person as well as those supporting and caring for them; thus there is a need for further research in an attempt to try to explain these experiences and increase our understanding of the dying process (Brayne et al., 2006; Ethier, 2005; Morse with Perry, 1994).

So what explanations have been put forward to account for these deathbed apparitions? One set of explanations proposes that these experiences are merely hallucinations brought on by, for example, an insufficient supply of oxygen to the brain cells (cerebral anoxia), brief disturbances of brain function, particularly in the temporal lobe regions, the presence of sedative or analgesic drugs, or they are brought on by stress or sensory deprivation (see Houran and Lange, 1997; McHarg, 1978, 1979: see reply by Haraldsson and Osis, 1979; Palmer, 1978; Turner, 1959). However, it has been argued that medication is not always a necessary requirement (see Houran and Lange, 1997), and some palliative care workers have asserted that normal drug-induced hallucinations are qualitatively different from deathbed apparition experiences (see Brayne et al., 2006). It is possible that the content of these deathbed experiences is influenced by patients' expectations about the dying process, particularly relating to their religion and culture (see Houran and Lange, 1997; Palmer, 1978) or their current needs (see Turner, 1959). An analysis of Barrett's case collection by Houran and Lange concluded that 'contextual variables [including cultural beliefs or expectations, situational demand characteristics, the emotional or physical state of the dying and embedded environmental cues] seem to play an important role in deathbed experiences because they provide perceptual structure for otherwise ambiguous dissociative or hallucinatory experiences' (1997: 1498) However, deathbed apparitions are also reported by those without any religious beliefs (see Grosso, 1981) and those who are unaware that they are dying (Barrett, 1926/1986). Osis and Haraldsson (1978: 398–9; 1986) also countered the claimed influence of expectations and beliefs and argued that, in their surveys, they found no relationship between patients' expectations and the identity and intentions of the reported deathbed apparitions. In addition, Barrett (1926/1986) noted that sometimes deathbed visions do not conform to patients' expectations; for example, a number of cases involved children who reported seeing angels but were puzzled because the angels did not seem to have any wings. More recent research among students enrolled in a death education course has also identified discrepancies between people's expectations of what a normal deathbed scene is like compared with reality (Kastenbaum and Normand, 1990). So, in summary, one normal explanation put forward for deathbed apparitions is that they are hallucinations whose content can be influenced by the context in which the dying persons find themselves as well as by their own personal beliefs and expectations. However, it is not entirely clear how all of the specific features common across many deathbed apparitions are thus created.

Alternatively, it has been suggested that deathbed apparition encounters involve paranormal processes or agents that are beyond our current scientific understanding. For example, in some cases the dying people apparently gain information, seemingly not through normal means of communication or logical inference, about the death of someone they did not know was dead (e.g., Hyslop, 1908; Houran and Lange, 1997; Myers, 1889: 24). Such information, as well as some of the alleged communication between the apparitions and the patients, or even between nursing staff and patients (Turner, 1959), might have an extrasensory perception (ESP) component to it (Bozzano, 1906; see Irwin and Watt, 2007). These experiences might consist of both real as well as imaginary elements (e.g., Betty, 2006). A traditional explanation for apparitions in general, as well as deathbed apparitions in particular (see Barrett, 1926/1986; Betty, 2006), is that they actually constitute some part of us – our spirit or soul or consciousness – that can survive bodily death. In fact, Osis and Haraldsson (1986: 7) consider deathbed observations to be a separate category of evidence for survival in their own right – in addition to mediumship, apparitions, reincarnation memories and out-of-body experiences (OBEs). However, Osis and Haraldsson's conclusions, based upon analyses of their own survey data, have been challenged on the grounds that other alternative explanations also fit the data equally well (e.g., McHarg, 1978; Palmer, 1978, 1979).

Irrespective of the ultimate explanation for these experiences, they do warrant further systematic scientific exploration, especially given the impact that they can have for the dying, their loved ones and health and social care practitioners. There is a need to compare fully the characteristics of dying people who do and do not report these kinds of deathbed experiences (see Hyslop, 1908: 107), as the latter group would provide a suitable control group. Rather than focusing attention on the features of the deathbed apparitions, there is also a need to pay more attention to the circumstances and context in which these experiences occur. Ultimately, we are striving for a theory that can explain all features of all cases and can make valid predictions about who is likely to have these experiences, with which particular features and in what circumstances. However, currently these deathbed experiences are not widely known about; public awareness should be increased and people need to be encouraged to share and discuss them with practitioners and researchers (see Brayne et al., 2006; Morse with Perry, 1994) so that people are in a better position to make sense of them, should they occur, and so that we can obtain sufficient data for future research.

References

Barrett, W. (1926/1986) *Death-bed Visions*. Wellingborough: Aquarian Press.

Betty, L. S. (2006) 'Are they hallucinations or are they real? The spirituality of deathbed and near-death visions', *Omega*, 53, 37–49.

Bozzano, E. (1906) 'Apparitions of deceased persons at death-beds', *The Annals of Psychical Science*, iii, 67–100.

Brayne, S., Farnham, C. and Fenwick, P. (2006) 'Deathbed phenomena and their effect on a palliative care team: A pilot study', *American Journal of Hospice & Palliative Medicine*, 23, 17–24.

Ethier, A. M. (2005) 'Death-related sensory experiences', *Journal of Pediatric Oncology Nursing*, 22, 104–111.

Giovetti, P. (1982) 'Near-death and deathbed experiences: an Italian survey', *Theta*, 10, 10–13.

Grosso, M. (1981) 'Toward an explanation of near-death phenomena', *Journal of the American Society for Psychical Research*, 75, 37–60.

Haraldsson, E. and Osis, K. (1979) [Letter], *Journal of the Society for Psychical Research*, 50, 126–8.

Houran, J. and Lange, R. (1997) 'Hallucinations that comfort: contextual mediation of deathbed visions', *Perceptual and Motor Skills*, 84, 1491–1504.

Hyslop, J. H. (1908) 'Visions of the dying', In *Psychical Research and the Resurrection*. London: Fisher Unwin. pp. 81–108.

Irwin, H. J. and Watt, C. A. (2007) *An Introduction to Parapsychology,* 5th edn. Jefferson, NC: McFarland.

Kastenbaum, R. and Normand, C. (1990) 'Deathbed scenes as imagined by the young and experienced by the old', *Death Studies*, 14, 201–17.

McHarg, J. F. (1978) 'At the hour of death by Karlis Osis and Erlendur Haraldsson' [Book Review], *Journal of the Society for Psychical Research*, 49, 885–7.

McHarg, J. F. (1979) [Letter], *Journal of the Society for Psychical Research*, 50, 128–9.

Morse, M. with Perry, P. (1994) *Parting Visions: An Exploration of Pre-death Psychic and Spiritual Experiences*. London: Piatkus.

Myers, F. W. H. (1889) 'On recognised apparitions occurring more than a year after death', *Proceedings of the Society for Psychical Research*, 6, 13–65.

Osis, K. (1961) *Deathbed Observations by Physicians and Nurses*. New York: Parapsychology Foundation.

Osis, K. and Haraldsson, E. (1978) Reply by Drs Osis and Haraldsson to Dr Palmer [Letter], *Journal of the American Society for Psychical Research*, 72, 395–400.

Osis, K. and Haraldsson, E. (1986) *At the Hour of Death* (revised edition). New York: Hastings House.

Palmer, J. (1978) 'Deathbed apparitions and the survival hypothesis' [Letter], *Journal of the American Society for Psychical Research*, 72, 392–5.

Palmer, J. (1979) 'More on deathbed apparitions and the survival hypothesis' [Letter], *Journal of the American Society for Psychical Research*, 73, 94–6.

Snell, J. (1928) *The Ministry of Angles: Here and Beyond*. London: Bell.

Turner, P. (1959) 'The grey lady: a study of a psychic phenomenon in the dying', *Journal of the Society for Psychical Research*, 40, 124–9.

79
Traveller Gypsies

Judith Okely

[...]

Interpretation

In referring to one aspect of the Gypsies' mortuary rites, Thompson suggests: 'Fear, then would seem to lie at the root of English Gypsy funeral Sacrifice' (1924: 89). But this is no explanation for the fear in the first place. Such an argument is tautologous. We should ask why the fear is so extreme among the Travellers. Although it might be argued by some that it is 'natural' for all peoples to feel frightened by the death of others, this does not explain why the Gypsies' beliefs and actions take these specific public forms. The Travellers' beliefs and actions cannot be explained away as 'common sense'. In some respects, they are markedly different from those of the surrounding Gorgios [the settled population]. Given that the Travellers regard themselves as different from Gorgios, it is also important to understand in what ways and why some of the Traveller's mortuary rites may be similar to those of the Gorgios.

First, at a Gypsy's death, the body is polluting and we see that attempts are made to place the dead in sanctified Gorgio territory. The outward appearance of the grave is kept orderly, although this attention cannot render the corpse clean and unpolluted. Recalling the vital separation for the Gypsies between the inner and outer body we see that in death the corpse and the *mulo* [ghost or spirit] are *mochadi* [ritually unclean or polluting]. This is because boundaries have been broken. First, at a Gypsy's death, I suggest, the separation between inner and outer body is no longer distinct; the inside has come outside. The corpse's clothes placed inside-out are a symbolic expression of this exposure. The bodily boundary is broken, so also is the boundary between Gypsy and Gorgio. It seems that the Travellers' tidying of the graves of their dead is in conformity with the Gorgios' emphasis on outer appearance, and in contrast to their priorities on their camp sites.

Secondly, there are also themes of settlement and appeasement in the Traveller's treatment of their dead. The Gorgio church service is treated as a *rite de passage* from the living and from the Gypsy group to an identity and place more Gorgio and settled. The grave in Gorgio hallowed ground is the necessary placing of the *mulo*, ideally sedentarised. It must not travel. Neither the polluted corpse nor parts of it must be allowed indecisive location. Hence the measures to prevent body snatching, dissection and transplants. Transplants would be doubly confusing as the organ would live on in another body. The dead body must be pinned down in space, just as Gorgios would pin down Gypsies on their sites.

The threat from the *mulo* is elaborate. It is not merely that it is polluted, it is also malevolent. What characteristics does the *mulo* possess? Its intentions cannot be known, it is unpredictable, it may hurt out of caprice. It may suddenly appear to the Gypsies and may as suddenly disappear. The *mulo* brings diseases and may try to lure Travellers to their death. It can sometimes be kept away if given its possessions and maybe food. Gypsies can more successfully outrun the *mulo* by travelling and avoiding places liked and frequented by it (cf. Sutherland 1975: 285).

I conclude that the *mulo* of a dead Gypsy has become like a Gorgio. Death is equivalent to assimilation. When the Travellers express their fear of the *mulo* they are reaffirming symbolically their fear of the Gorgio. Like the *mulo*, the Gorgio is unpredictable and may suddenly enter a camp site and as quickly disappear. The Gorgio may hurt or prosecute out of caprice. The Gorgio is *mochadi*, brings diseases and lures Gypsies to their death. The Gorgio in a sedentary society has a permanent interest in property. Just as the Travellers must avoid the favourite camp sites of their dead, so the Travellers must avoid land which Gorgios have regularly frequented. To escape Gorgio control, the Gypsies appear to give Gorgios what they want. To appease the *mulo*, the Gypsies give wreaths and attention, and abandon claims to its property. Gorgios must be discouraged from entering the trailer, and as with the *mulo*, elaborate devices are used to keep them out. If the Gorgio, like the *mulo*, cannot be kept at a distance by discouraging intimacy, the Gypsies keep traveling.

In some discussions the Travellers consciously associate banishment or assimilation with death. When a Traveller is banished from the group, the father and family pronounce the Traveller dead. His or her name is never mentioned again and is seen as polluting. This may happen when a Gypsy 'marries out' and to a Gorgio specifically disapproved of by the Gypsies, or when the Gypsy has committed an outrageous act.

> When a Gypsy woman ran off with a married Gypsy man she left her children, whom her deserted husband put into a Gorgio home as revenge. The woman's father was informed and, to his humiliation, had to collect them. The father threatened to 'cry dead' his daughter. 'That'd been a terrible thing. He would never 've talked of her again. He wouldn't have gone to her funeral 'cos she'd be already dead. But he took pity on the grandchildren.'

In these circumstances the Gypsy is obliged to move into Gorgio society, and banishment is equated with death. Other forms of assimilation are associated with death: after the new 'permanent' and Gorgio conrolled sites were opened, the Travellers' anxiety was indicated by their comments on the number of deaths which had occurred among tenants. 'There's several Travellers who 'ave died since these sites were opened. Something's wrong.' In fact the more elaborate sites tended to attract the aged and infirm, but this explanation for one or two deaths on sites was not suggested. Instead, the sites were seen as inherently threatening.

In the cases above, assimilation is equated with death, but I am also arguing the inverse: that death is less explicitly equated with assimilation or even sedentarisation, given the Gypsies' ideology of travelling. When the Gypsies destroy a dead person's property they are reminding themselves that complex inheritance laws and accumulated property are associated with sedentarisation. Extra special observances are required of close kin in laying the *mulo* to rest, to show that they do not benefit, through inheritance, by their cognate's death. They also demonstrate to the rest of the community that they have disassociated themselves from the dead.

Funerals, however, are not merely the concern of close cognates, [...]. Any Travellers acquainted with the deceased gather together to dispatch the dead Gypsy from the living. The unity of Gypsies at funerals, transcending internal rivalry, is both a political and religious statement. All Travellers must combine against the greater threat of death within the group and against the Gorgio, whose likeness Gypsies assume after death. The Gorgio pursues the Gypsies to the grave and at the grave.

I saw how the police provided an escort for a Gypsy funeral procession: not, the Gypsies stated, for traffic control, but to trap a man on the run, who must surely attend. He did, and everyone knew. The Gypsies rejoiced that he came and went free.

Thus there seems no joyful beyond, no Gypsy survival after death, only a blank space; a nothingness to be filled by Gorgios. The ultimate truth is that Gypsies are not separated from Gorgios in death. For Travellers, their children are their regeneration; the continuous thread of existence. Their dead ancestors are not the focus of continuity. As a revengeful and unpredictable *mulo,* the dead individual loses Gypsy or Traveller identity and his or her name is written in a Gorgio medium on the gravestone. The dead Traveller is no longer classified as a member of the Gypsy group which continues elsewhere, in another place. In the celebrated 'Wind on the Heath' dialogue the Gypsy Jasper Petulengro says: 'When a man dies, he is cast into the earth, and there is an end of the matter.' Petulengro argues with Borrow:

> 'Life is very sweet, brother; who would wish to die?'
> 'I would wish to die…'
> 'You talk like a gorgio – which is the same as talking like a fool – were you a Romany Chal you would talk wiser. Wish to die, indeed!… A Romany Chal would wish to live for ever!'
>
> (Borrow, 1851: 325–6)

Acceptance of death is thus treated as a Gorgio characteristic.

Thus we see that so-called 'resurrectionism' and the Travellers' use of Gorgio church and graveyards are neither raw material for nor evidence of conversion to the Gorgio brand of Christianity. The Gypsies' mortuary rites are neither merely 'magical beliefs' as has been patronisingly suggested (Trigg 1968: 100), nor admirable piety. As in many mortuary rites, the identity, social organisation and ideology of the living are disguised and inverted. That which pleases the Gorgio observer is ironically a rejection of his or her kind. The boundary between life and death is used to make symbolic statements about another ethnic boundary. The loss of a Gypsy through death is not seen merely as a loss of another human being and member of an amorphous society, but the loss of a member of a specific minority group, always vulnerable within the larger society. The Gypsy dead have crossed the ethnic boundary. The mortuary rites affirm the living Gypsies' separation from Gorgios, and their fear of becoming one of them.

References

Borrow, G. (1851) *Lavengro.* London: Murray.
Sutherland, A. (1975) *Gypsies: the Hidden Americans.* London: Tavistock.
Thompson, T. W. (1924) English Gypsy Death and Burial Customs. *J.G.L.S.,* third series, vol. II (1–2) 5–38, 60–93.
Trigg, E. B. (1968) Religion and Social Reform among the Gysies of Britain. *J.G.L.S.*, third series, vol. XLVII (3–4) 82–109.

Also see Okely, J. (2008) 'Knowing without Notes', in N. Halstead, E. Hirsch and J. Okely (eds), *Knowing How to Know*. Oxford: Berghahn.

80

If the Spirit Moves You

Justine Picardie

[...]

Number 33 houses the Spiritualist Association of Great Britain. I've been thinking about coming here for months now, ever since a friend of mine told me that daily demonstrations of mediumship take place at 3.30 every weekday afternoon. Today seems as good a day as any to visit this place ... no, more than that, today must be the best day of the year to come. As I push open the big black front door, I'm excited again; the same way I felt as a child on my way to a friend's birthday party (and I've come here for a social gathering of the dead, I suppose). The lady at the reception desk takes my entrance fee – £4 – and points me towards the sweeping staircase. 'It's on the first floor, dear,' she says, 'through the door on your left.'

Inside the upstairs room, which is in half-darkness as the curtains are still drawn, there are many rows of flip-up seats – a hundred or more, as if in a cinema. I take one near the front, beside a notice on the wall which says: 'This Hall Is Named In Memory of Sir Oliver Lodge FRS – a great leader in physical and pyschic research.' It's a good omen, I decide – because Lodge was not only the inventor of the spark plug, but also cited by Judith Chisholm as a forerunner in the search for a scientific means to communicate with the dead.

There are three old ladies in the audience, and two grey-haired men. One more woman arrives, wheezing deeply, and sits beside me. She is wearing a pink hat clamped to her head, and a pink coat, over a pink velour track suit, with mauve appliqué flowers on the front. I would guess she is in her eighties.

The medium appearing here today is called Julie Johnson. She, too, is wearing a pink top – though her outfit is more muted than my neighbour's (neat tweed skirt, tan tights, flat black shoes, sensible sweater). She stands on the raised platform at the end of the room, and opens the curtains behind her. 'There, I'll let in the light,' she says, cheerfully. There is a grand piano to one side of her, and a lectern in front, between two large, elaborate flower arrangements of the type one might find in a church. I study the flowers, trying to work out whether they're real or fake, but it's hard to tell (one moment I'm so convinced they're real that I'm sure I can smell the scent of decay coming from the vases; the next, I can almost see the dust on the fabric leaves.) Julie talks quickly to us, offering up a prayer of peace and harmony in the same brisk tones that a chairwoman of the WI might give thanks to a visiting speaker. 'I'm just the telephone between you and your spirits,' says Julie. 'But I can hear them, see them, sometimes even smell them'.

She half closes her eyes – and, for a moment, I think she looks like a blind person – and when she opens them, she points to a stony-faced woman on the other side of the room to me. The woman is wearing black. 'I can see a cuddly, homely looking lady in the spirit world,' says Julie to the women. 'She has a velvety red chair, and she crochets bits and pieces for her home. It must be lovely to be able to make such nice things. Oh, and she keeps her house very tidy, very neat. Does that mean anything to you?'

The woman in black nods, though her face is still immobile. 'Now I see you riding donkeys on a beach with this lady,' says Julie. 'Ah, happy days … you had such fun. Does that mean anything to you?' The woman nods again, though this time her face is melting. 'She loves you very much,' says Julie. 'She's your auntie, isn't she?' Two tears run down the woman's face, and I can't stop myself looking at her, but when she sees my face turned in her direction, I feel embarrassed, and stare at the ceiling, as if I'm looking for guidance in the crystal chandelier. There are large damp patches on the ceiling, as if all the tears cried in this room have risen towards the sky, but somehow got caught up in the plaster instead.

Then Julie turns to me. My turn! I sit up straight, excited again, concentrating on the memory of Ruth's smile, willing her to make a dramatic appearance today – it's Halloween, for God's sake – right here in Belgrave Square. 'I see your grandfather,' says Julie, 'your mother's father.'

'Oh,' I say, feeling faintly disappointed.

'He's showing me all his plans and documents and papers,' she says. 'Was he a lawyer?'

'No,' I say, trying not to sound truculent, 'a civil engineer.'

'Well, he's worried about Timothy,' says Julie. 'Does that mean anything to you?' As a matter of fact, it does. Timothy is my mother's twin brother, though she never speaks about him, or to him. She has said, occasionally, that he was their parents' favourite, but nothing very much more than that.

The Timothy reference is rather impressive, but even so, I'm disappointed – where's Ruth in all of this? But Julie has moved on again, and I'm catching snippets of other people's stories, other people's spirits. It's like listening to someone else's incomprehensible dreams – though the details are familiar; the stuff of domestic life, rather than gothic tales of death. Julie tells the lady in pink beside me that the spirits know she's been worried about the guttering outside her house. 'But don't worry, you're going to get it sorted out, and you can use that chap who's already given you a quote for the job. He's cheap – and he's very trustworthy.'

After dealing with the building problems of the lady in pink, Julie turns her attention to the anxious-looking grey-haired man behind me. 'I can see a spirit sitting right beside you, sir,' she says, 'and from the look of him, he's your father.' A small smile lights up the man's face. 'Your father says you've got a hobby that you could turn into a job,' continues Julie. 'You've been feeling a bit down – a bit betrayed, almost, at work – but your father says, don't worry, everything is going to turn out fine.'

These homely ghosts continue to dish out soothing advice – about haircuts, travel arrangements, new houses, holidays. It's the kind of chat that my mother's parents were so good at – quiet, gentle homilies that came with milky tea and digestive biscuits. My grandparents would feel at home here, I think, if they were to feel at home anywhere in his noisy world. Maybe I should listen out for their soft lost voices more often … instead of allowing my longing for Ruth to drive everyone else from my head?

After an hour, Julie draws the meeting to a close, and thanks us and our attendant spirits for being here today. She leaves at an anxious trot, muttering about her next appointment, and I'm half-tempted to run after her, and ask for more; to follow her in case she knows the way to slip through a wrinkle in time; a secret rabbit hole that leads to the wonderland of the dead. […]

81
Is Anybody There?

Jo Dawson

When my Nan died in the autumn of 2000, the last thing on my mind was seeing if I could get in touch with her on 'the other side'. Whilst I was, and still am, convinced that there is an afterlife, I certainly didn't want to confirm that was the case by chasing her to tie-up loose ends. This wasn't the case though for other members of my family. Over the course of the next few months, various female relatives sought solace and comfort in their grief by making one last contact with her through a spiritualist.

Whilst my Nan had been ill with tuberculosis during her last few months, no one really expected it to claim her life. No one sought out a final opportunity to say goodbyes, to tell her that they loved her, to ask the unanswered questions that for some continued to haunt them when she was gone.

My aunt is the third child of four daughters. She was the main carer for my Nan and my Granddad during their final months. She and her husband took the responsibility for ensuring that the food shopping was done, that my Granddad, who is disabled, received the medical attention he needed, and responding to the many, and often what seemed to be irritating and trivial, requests – 'Can you come and draw the curtains for me' was one of the requests, which involved a 20-minute journey there and back again. In many ways, she was the one family member who did the most for my Nan during that time, and yet after her death she was overwhelmed by a sense of failure, of not having done enough. She and her husband moved in to care for my Granddad, abandoning their own comfortable home. Yet still my aunt felt she had somehow let my Nan down. And so she sought the expertise and the skills of 'Jenny', a local and renowned spiritualist, to get in touch with my Nan and check that she was OK.

This communication resolved many outstanding issues in my aunt's mind. My aunt asked, had she done enough? Should she have done more? Had she let her down in those final months? Jenny assured her that my Nan didn't feel this was the case, she had done everything and more than she would have wanted or expected. But was this really a communication from the beyond the grave, or was Jenny merely telling my aunt what she wanted to hear?

The session concluded with one last message from my Nan; a message that those of us who knew her didn't find in the least surprising. My aunt was admonished by my Nan for leaving the cups to drain rather than drying them up immediately. How could Jenny have known that my Nan had been a stickler for drying up as soon as the washing-up had been done and would never have tolerated leaving the cups to drain?

The sense of closure that my aunt achieved from this session led to her daughter visiting the same spiritualist. I'm not sure exactly what she was seeking from this session, but she did want to have something to remember my Nan by. Jenny described a ring and told her that my Nan wanted her, one of four granddaughters, to have that particular ring. As she sorted through my Nan's jewellery that night with her mother and my Granddad, she found a ring exactly as described amongst the items.

Interestingly enough, the next relative to seek contact was not a blood relative of my Nan's, it was her granddaughter-in-law. Julie had married my cousin, after 10 years together, in the July before my Nan died. It had been the last family celebration when we had all been together and was the last time many relatives saw my Nan alive. Julie had been very close to my Nan, who often told her she was too good for my cousin! She also seemed to delight in telling her that they had left it too late to get married and have children – this was her way of encouraging them up the aisle. She was overjoyed at their wedding and despite claiming she couldn't afford all the great-grandchildren that were appearing, it was obvious she couldn't wait for a child to be born to this marriage. When my Nan died, Julie became convinced that my Nan had been right and she would never have the children she so desperately longed for. This conviction grew as the longed-for pregnancy never materialised.

Six months after my Nan's death, Julie visited Margaret, a medium who promised to obtain the answers she was seeking. My Nan told Margaret that she felt Julie's husband was not looking after her and she was, as always, too good for him. Then Julie asked the two-million dollar question of Margaret and my Nan – had she left it too late to have children? The answer was swift and determined – no she hadn't; she would indeed have the baby she wanted so badly. Julie was over-joyed at this news and seemed to find new vigour. But, as the months turned into years and there was still no pregnancy she began to doubt what she had been told. Had Margaret told her what she wanted to hear? Was it all a sham? Did she really make contact?

Seven years after my Nan died, Julie gave birth to her much-longed for baby. The baby that my Nan told her she would have from beyond the grave.

My question remains: Is anybody there? Ask these three members of my family and the resounding answer is: Yes! Ask me, who witnessed it from the sidelines, and my answer remains: 'I don't know and I don't intend on finding out for myself!'

82

Experience of the Loss of a Husband/Father

Dorothy Thornton and Gayle Letherby

How and when it happened

When my husband Ron died I was 47. He was seven and a half years older than me, and we had a daughter Gayle who had just had her 20th birthday three weeks before. We had been married for 22 years and in all that time I had never known Ron to have to go to the doctor.

Living in a village in Cornwall, Ron and I worked in the tourist industry in the summer. In the winter of 1978/79 we were renting a house from an elderly friend and Ron was doing some decorating for her. One day in January it was very cold and windy, so when Gayle had left for college we shut ourselves in and Ron started to paint. Towards lunchtime he said that he had indigestion, so I said 'Why don't you go and have a rest and I'll finish the painting and then we can have a hot drink and something to eat.' A little later I went upstairs to see how Ron was and he was lying still on the floor. I knew it must be something serious, and as we didn't have a phone I ran over the road to a friend's house and asked her to ring for an ambulance. I ran back to Ron. I knew he was dead. I put a blanket over him, knelt on the floor and put my arms around him. It seemed like ages but at last a paramedic ran into the room. I said 'He is dead, isn't he?' hoping that he would say 'no', but instead he said 'Go downstairs, send the other paramedic up and we will do what we can'. Soon they came down and said that they were sorry, but there was nothing they could do. Just then our doctor, who my friend had also telephoned, came running up the hill to our house. He and I went upstairs to Ron and he said that there would have to be a post-mortem as it was a sudden death. He asked if there was anyone who could come and stay with me and I said that my daughter would be home soon. He offered to ring the school where Gayle was doing her college placement, say that her dad was ill and ask if someone could bring her home to me. I didn't want him to do that as I thought she would guess what had happened, but he said it was best that she come home before they came to take Ron away.

Finding out

In my second placement of my nursery nurse training at an infant's school 12 miles away from home, I was sticking the children's pictures on the classroom walls and half-listening to the teacher read a story to her class of 7-year-olds when the head-teacher walked into the classroom and with little pre-amble told me that my father had been taken ill. I could never remember my father being really ill, a cold or two of course, some pain following trips to the dentist, but nothing more serious than that. So at that moment I knew, just knew that he was dead. The journey home passed in a blur; the teacher was kind but clumsily asked questions that only confirmed what I already knew; 'How old is your father, Gayle?' being just one.

The first evening and the next few days

After the doctor had left I went outside to wait for Gayle. When I saw her coming up the hill I went to meet her and told her that her father had died. 'I will take care of you, mum', she said; 'We will take care of each other, we are on our own now', I replied. We went into the house and together we went to see Ron before they took him away. Then we sat and talked about what we had to do. Gayle rang her boyfriend who was at University in London and I rang a close friend of Ron's, and they both said they would come the next day. The next few days we were busy making all the arrangements. I went to the bank to have Ron's, bank account closed and for the first time took out a bank account in my own name. Whilst busily doing all of the things we had to do, I began to feel angry with Ron for going away and leaving us on our own. I thought daft, stupid things such as 'he should be here helping to do all of this'.

The funeral

My dad's funeral was always going to be different, because my dad was different. In order to follow his dreams, our small family left Liverpool, the home of all our births, in the mid-1960s and travelled for several years – around the British Isles and abroad – before settling back in England, in Cornwall. Because of my father's sense of adventure our lives were rather different than most; transient and sometimes insecure, yet interesting and always full of love. There were other ways in which he made his mark too, and these had an impact on the way in which we said our goodbyes. The first thing he would do when waking up in the morning was push back the curtains to let in the sunshine, so there was no way that my mum or I were going to close the curtains on the morning of his funeral 'in respect of the dead' as is convention. Neither were we going to wear black or anything drab. He would have hated that. He liked his 'girls' to look good. I remember as a small child my mum and I used to line up for 'inspection' before a family day out. So we wore his favourites of our clothes proudly to church. Reading back this paragraph my father sounds controlling, but it's important to remember that my father was a man of his time; born in 1923 it's not surprising that he saw himself as 'the man of the house'. Man of the house he was, but a loving, gentle, fun-loving patriarch I'd say.

During the service it was clear that the vicar had taken the time to find out many things about Ron (not Ronald or Ronnie, both of which he hated) even though he had not spoken in detail to my mother or me about my dad. This of course brought my mum and I great comfort as it indicated the high regard my father was held in by others in our village; the village that he'd loved for years but only lived in for nine months.

The next few months and years

After the funeral Gayle and I slowly began to get on with our lives. Gayle said she would postpone her wedding, due to take place in June of the same year, but I encouraged her to carry on with her original plans. After she was married she went to live in London and I carried on working in a hotel in the village. Gayle came to see me as often as she could, and after the summer season each year I would go and spend a few weeks with her and her husband.

Dreams and regrets

A couple of years after his death I dreamt of my father. He was standing with a group of other men; tall, dark and strong, dressed in smart trousers and a bright white shirt. He looked just as I remembered him. 'He's an angel' I thought, which was not – I think – a reflection of religious feelings and beliefs but an acknowledgement of my dad as a special person, someone who my friends of that time still regularly talk of with affection and admiration.

Nearly 29 years on, my life, not surprisingly, is very different than it was in the late 1970s. My first husband and I divorced in the early 1990s and I've since married again. After practising as a nursery nurse for several years, I entered higher education as a mature student in the late 1980s (see Letherby in Part V). Since then I've pursued a career in academia. Like everyone, my life is peppered with problems and pleasures, losses and triumphs. Over the years I've found that I miss my dad the most at the good times: I'm sad he's missed meeting my new partner and new friends, regret that I've been unable to share achievements with him, and miss so much his expressions of love and pride. I miss him as I contribute to this piece.

Us now

We were always a close family; Ron believing that Gayle and I were 'the best things since sliced bread'. I've never married again, never wanted another partner after Ron. But I have a good life. I'm retired now and live in a small market town a few miles away from the village where Ron, Gayle and I lived. I like living on my own and my own company but I'm often away, visiting or travelling with Gayle. We are even closer than we were when Ron was alive, and friends regularly comment on the closeness of our relationship. She has done what she said she would do on the day that Ron died and has always looked after me, and I do what I can for her. I was quite young when Ron died but he left me with a wonderful daughter, and I like to think that wherever he is now he knows that we are OK.

83

Sparkling Epitaphs: From Jewels to Web Portraits, We've Moved On from the Tombstone

Roger Dobson

The bright yellow precious stone on Sandra Wilson's necklace is not the usual sort of diamond. It's made from the ashes of her 11-year-old son Rhodri, who died from a rare blood disorder.

After cremation, carbon was extracted from his ashes and converted into the £12,000, one-carat diamond on the necklace she is wearing. "I thought it would be a bit morbid having the usual memorial and I wanted something that would be there permanently, and which could be passed down from generation to generation," she says. "We collected the ashes and the company sent them off to America where the carbon from his ashes was processed for five months, using heat and compression, and turned into this beautiful diamond. I've just got it back and I wear it constantly. It has helped the grieving because it is a reminder of my son."

Wilson is among an increasing number of people in Britain who have preserved the ashes of loved ones in the form of LifeGem diamonds. She is also part of a wider trend, where people seek new ways of celebrating and recording the deaths of relatives and friends.

[...] Not only is death being marked differently, with the rise of roadside memorials, green funerals and postmortem portraits, but there is also a different attitude to death. A century ago, views were shaped by a fervent belief in Heaven and Hell. The decline of religion, social changes and the rise of science have altered our beliefs about death and afterlife. We still believe (or want to believe) that there is an afterlife, but we acknowledge that whatever it is, it's more subtle than previously thought.

"If you look at the research, belief in Hell has virtually disappeared from the Western world, apart from in America and Ireland. Belief in resurrection of the body has taken a tumble, too," says Tony Walter, a reader in sociology at Reading University. "When I ask my students about this kind of thing, a lot of them tick the box for an eternal soul but hardly anyone ticks the box for a resurrected body, although there is still a strong desire to believe that something of us continues."

Cremation has also changed the way we regard death. With burials and tombstones, the dead occupied the same physical realm as the living. Cremations changed all that, raising questions

---

Roger Dobson, 'Sparkling epitaphs: From jewels to web portraits, we've moved on from the tombstone', *The Times*, September 10th, www.timesonline.co.uk/tol/life_and_style/health/features/article564339.ece.

about whether the dead exist any more. Research suggests that one of the main anxieties about death is a fear of being forgotten or ignored. We might accept that the body doesn't make it to the afterlife but social immortality, the need to be remembered, is still needed. Jennifer Crew Solomon, of Winthrop University, South Carolina, says her research suggests that this is increasingly being achieved by giving gifts to people in the belief that they will remember the deceased. But, she warns that the road to social immortality has it pitfalls: "we found the process did not always go smoothly. Several family members may, for example, want the same item."

Along with immortality, death's sting seems to have abated somewhat, too. One Dutch study suggests that people are more comfortable with the idea of mortality, thanks to television and celebrity deaths. Anton Kos, of the Zuiderzee Museum in the Netherlands, says: "Television series such as *Six Feet Under* enjoy a huge audience and funeral ceremonies of celebrities have contributed to a more open mind regarding death and burial, and especially one's own death. The fear of death has not vanished but most people seem to be more comfortable with it, which explains why so many are eager to arrange their own funeral."

About 10,000 people a year have non-religious funerals in Britain and that figure is growing by 20 per cent a year. Natural burials and DIY ceremonies are increasing too, says Josefine Speyer, the co-founder of the Natural Death Centre. "People who choose to organise a funeral without the help of a funeral director often do so because it allows them to create a life-celebratory event that is individual and meaningful, and allows them to have control at a time when they feel a lack of control." But the biggest area of change has been in the way we record and celebrate the lives of loved ones and it is the baby-boomers who are leading demand for more personalised deaths.

George Dickinson, a researcher of the College of Charleston, and an expert in personalised death trends, predicts that traditional interment ceremonies and graveyards may soon be dead and buried. "One option for remembering the dead is a fingerprint-impression keepsake of the deceased. A ring can be also made from the gold in the deceased person's teeth and remains can be put into a painting or placed in orbit."

Or you could follow the lead of the late author Hunter S. Thompson whose last spectacular gesture involved having his ashes packed into a specially commissioned firework and fired from a cannon to a height of 500ft above the Rocky Mountains last month.

The decline in the traditional burial and gravestone has also resulted in a drop in the popularity of the epitaph. Gravestones are more likely to carry pictures of the deceased than important words. But that could be about to change, with the arrival of the e-pitaph. Give an internet site a list of the people you love or hate, and on the day of your death, e-mails will be sent out telling them exactly what you thought of them.

Index